This book is a donation from
Dr. Ivory Nelson,
President
Central Washington
University.

THE SKIPPER'S INSTANT HELPER

Also by ERNEST A. ZADIG

A HANDBOOK OF MODERN MARINE MATERIALS

THE COMPLETE BOOK OF BOAT ENGINES

THE COMPLETE BOOK OF BOAT ELECTRONICS

THE COMPLETE BOOK OF BOATING

INVENT AND GET RICH

FUNDAMENTALS OF AIR CONDITIONING

plus numerous magazine articles

THE SKIPPER'S INSTANT HELPER

ERNEST A. ZADIG

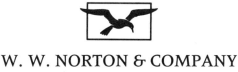

W. W. Norton & Company

NEW YORK   LONDON

Copyright © 1992 by Ernest A. Zadig.
All rights reserved. Printed in the United States of America.
First Edition

The text of this book is composed in Meridien
with the display set in Meridien Medium
Composition by University Graphics
Manufacturing by Vail Ballou
Book design by Jacques Chazaud

Library of Congress Cataloging-in-Publication Data
Zadig, Ernest A., 1899–
   The skipper's instant helper / Ernest A. Zadig.
      p.   cm.

   1. Boats and boating—Equipment and supplies—Handbooks, manuals,
etc.   2. Yachts and yachting—Equipment and supplies—Handbooks,
manuals, etc.   I. Title.
VM321.Z33   1992
623.8′223′028—dc20   92-10414

     ISBN 0-393-03341-4

W.W. Norton & Company, Inc., 500 Fifth Avenue, New York, N.Y. 10110
W.W. Norton & Company, Ltd., 10 Coptic Street, London WC1A 1PU

1 2 3 4 5 6 7 8 9 0

To
AUDREY
and to
JANE

About the Author

Ernest A. Zadig has been a boatman "since way back." By profession an engineer, he has been appointed Author-in-Residence emeritus by the Florida Institute of Technology; he is also an Adjunct Professor emeritus. He holds numerous patents in various fields, and has owned and operated an electronics manufacturing plant. He is the author of a series of successful boating books.

His home is an 85-foot twin-diesel yacht. Among the onboard features of the ship are a complete workshop, a photographic dark room, and an electronics laboratory.

Foreword

The Skipper's Instant Helper is a selection of 150 items of boat ownership and use that often confuse skippers. This book should help to clear up such confusion. The text is arranged alphabetically for easy finding.

The text in each section is divided into various parts. First is a complete technical description, in layman's language, of design and construction, functioning and use. "Installation" and "Maintenance" outline recommended installation and maintenance procedures. Where applicable, "Troubleshooting" details logical troubleshooting, and "Repair" explains repairs within the ability of the average boatman.

Illustrations are captioned under the same heading as that of the text they explain. Many photographs and special drawings are used.

Referrals throughout the text direct the reader to related subjects and additional information that should further aid his understanding.

May *The Skipper's Instant Helper* iron out the wrinkles that can lessen the fun of boating.

Ernest A. Zadig
Florida Institute of Technology
Melbourne, Florida, 1991

Contents

Airconditioning 11
Alarms 13
Alternators 14
Amplifier Symbols 16
Anchoring 17
Anchors 19
Antennas 22
Autopilots 24
Barometers 27
Batteries 27
Bedding Compounds 30
   (Elastomerics)
Bench Tests 32
Bilge Blowers 33
Bilge Pumps 33
Bilge Switches 34
Binoculars 35
Blocks 36
Block Diagrams 38
Bow Thrusters 38
Bowden Wires 40
Breaker Points 40
Capacitors 41
Carburetors 42
Cavitation 45
Chargers 45
Chocks 46
Circuit Breakers 46
Cleats 47
Compasses 48
Control Cables 50
Crash Pads 51
Cruising Hazards 51
Davits 54
Deadrise 55
Depthsounders 55

Diesel Fuel 58
Diodes 59
Direction Finders 60
   (RDFS)
Displacement/Planning 62
Doppler Effect 63
Dynamometers 63
Electricity 64
Electrolysis 67
Electronic Control 69
Emergency Gear 70
Engine Overheating 71
Engines 71
EPIRBs 75
Fiberglass 76
Filters (Fuel) 80
Fire Extinguishers 82
Fluxgate Compasses 84
Fuel Pumps 86
Fuses 86
Generator Sets 86
Grounds 88
Gyro Compasses 91
Hauling Out 91
Heads 94
Heat Sinks 96
Holding Tanks 97
Hose Safety 98
Hydraulic Steering 98
Hydrometers 99
Ignition 99
Inflatables 102
Insurance 104
Integrating/Interfacing 105
Inverters 105
Jet Drives 106

CONTENTS

Knotmeters 106
Lead Lines 108
Life Rails 108
Lightning Rods 109
Loran-C 110
Lubricating Oils 112
Maneuvering Boards 113
Mildew 114
Navigation Lights 114
Navigation Markers 118
Night Boating 120
Outboard Motors 120
Paints 122
Personal Flotation Devices 126
Plotting 128
Polarity (Electric) 128
Preamplifiers 129
Propellers 130
Radar Reflectors 132
Radars 132
Ranges 134
Refrigeration 136
Rope Cutter 137
Rope Starters 138
Rudder Indicators 139
Rudders 139
Rules of the Road 140
Rust 141
Sails 142
Satellite Navigation Systems 144
Sea Anchors 146
Seacocks 147
Seagoing Clocks 148
Self-Steerers 148
Shore Cables 150
Single Sideband 151
Soldering 153
Spark Plugs 155
Spring Lines 157
Stabilizers 158
Standing Wave Ratio 160

Starters 161
Static 163
Steering Torque 164
Stern-Drives 165
Stoves 167
Strobe Lights 168
Stuffing Boxes 169
Synchronizers 169
Tachometers 170
Thermostats 170
Tides and Currents 171
Tilt/Trim 173
Transducers 175
Transformers 176
Transistors 177
Transmissions 178
Trim Tabs 181
Trouble Lamps 182
TV Afloat 184
Universal Joints 184
Vapor Alarms 184
Variable-Ratio Oiling 186
Varnishes 186
Vectors 188
Ventilation Systems 188
VHF-FM Radios 189
Video Charts 191
Voltage Regulators 193
Volt and Ampere Meters 193
Voltohmmeters (VOM) 195
Water Purifiers 196
Water Tanks 197
Watt Meters 197
Weather 198
Winches 200
Wind/Current vs. Course 202
Wire Rope 203
Wire Splices 204
Wiring Code 204
Zincs 207

AIRCONDITIONING

Airconditioning

Airconditioning has become an almost universal comfort on cabin pleasure boats large and small. Cooling equipment designed for marine use is commonly installed by the boatbuilder, or else it is purchased in the aftermarket and placed aboard by the owner.

Operation of an airconditioner demands electric current far beyond the ability of boat batteries to supply. Thus, there are two choices: either have airconditioned comfort only at the pier from the marina pier line, or add an adequate generator set (see Generator Sets) for cooling underway or at anchor.

The cooling power of an airconditioning unit is rated in Btus and/or in tons. One ton is equivalent to 12,000 Btus. Equipment labeled "one ton" can deliver the same cooling as can one ton of ice melting in 24 hours. A rough overview shows small cabin boats with half-ton (airconditioning) installations and large cruisers with cooling capabilities rising into the multi-tons.

The undesired heat extracted from a living space may be dissipated into the ambient outside air (air to air), or it may be thrust into the surrounding water (water to air). The latter method has advantages and it is more efficient—but it also has a drawback, as noted below in the discussion on condensers.

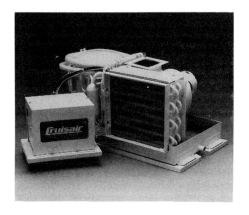

AIRCONDITIONING—This self-contained airconditioning system transfers the heat from the cabin to the surrounding water. Reverse-cycle operation takes heat from the sea and provides cabin warmth for cool days. Remember that a through-hull fitting and pump are required for cooling the condenser with Sea water (water to air). *(Courtesy Marine Development Corp.)*

An airconditioning system consists of an alternating-current (AC) electric motor-driven compressor, a condenser, a refrigerant flow control, an evaporator, and various filters and driers. The flow control may be a capillary tube, a thermostatic expansion valve, or an automatic expansion valve. The fluid that circulates inside the system is a fluorocarbon called Freon, chosen for its efficient vaporizing and condensing.

AIRCONDITIONING

The operating cycle starts at the compressor that puts the Freon under pressure and forces it to the condenser, where it arrives as a hot gas. The cooling effect of the condenser causes the hot gas to change to a liquid. The condenser either is air cooled by reason of multiple fins or it is water cooled. The water-cooled type is a tube within a tube, one for the gas and the other for the circulating water, supplied by a seawater pump.

The water-cooled condenser is more efficient and much less bulky, but, as mentioned earlier, it has a drawback: fouling and clogging by seawater organisms and vegetation. In Florida, for example, barnacles enter while in almost a microscopic stage and find conditions excellent for growth to a size that impedes water flow and stops the system.

The flow of Freon from the condenser to the evaporator is controlled either by a capillary tube, by a thermostatic expansion valve, or by an automatic expansion valve. Of these, the capillary tube is the simplest, being merely a length of small-bore metal tubing. The rate of Freon flow determines the rate at which cooling is taking place.

The evaporator is kept under lowered pressure by the sucking action of the compressor intake. When liquid Freon is allowed to enter by the control, it immediately flashes into a gas. This change of state from liquid to vapor is the heart of the cooling action, because it cannot take place without the addition of heat. This heat is extracted from the living space that is being cooled. A blower forces room air over the cold fins of the evaporator.

The suction intake of the compressor withdraws the expanded Freon from the evaporator, and the cycle is repeated endlessly.

Airconditioning units for pleasure boats are sold as complete packages housed in a cabinet or framework. Those with water-cooled condensers have greater latitude for placement beacause a seawater pump removes the need for wide air circulation. (Of course, the evaporator blower must still be located to circulate cooled living-space air.)

Installation The seawater pump for the condenser may be either positive-displacement or centrifugal. The former may be placed in the bilge above the waterline, the latter slightly below the waterline. The addition of a cleanable filter with a transparent body is advisable for frequent clean-out of fouling. Pumps with magnetic drive are preferred, because this eliminates the seals that are a frequent cause of leakage.

The airconditioning installation may also be made in split fashion, with the evaporator and its blower in the living space and the balance of the machinery elsewhere (for instance, in the bilge). The connection would be two insulated lines of copper tubing, the suction line and the liquid line. The seawater pump is wired in parallel with the compressor motor and runs whenever the unit is in use. The evaporator blower motor is under separate control, preferably multi-speed.

Maintenance Maintenance concerns itself with keeping the fins of the evaporator clean and checking for fouling of the seawater filter. A thermometer in the output air of the evap-

ALARMS

orator should register approximately 10 degrees Fahrenheit below the temperature of room air. There should be no frost on the suction line. The liquid line should be very warm.

Repair Airconditiong repair would be within the ability of a handy skipper were it not for the tools and instruments required to do the job. Hence, the usual option is a repair call to a technician.

Alarms

Electronic alarms are automatic watchmen that relieve the skipper's anxiety for his boat both at dock and at sea. The alarms warn of trouble within, such as lubrication or coolant stoppage, and they warn of trouble from without, such as unauthorized entry and burglary. The equipment is simple in the extreme, consisting of various forms of normally open and normally closed switches. A relay is added to prevent an intruder from silencing the bell or horn by immediate closure of the entry means.

A more complicated alarm device monitors explosive vapors and is a prime safety feature for all gasoline-operated boats. While the human nose is an excellent vapor detector, a robot sniffer constantly on watch is a great reassurance.

Specifically, alarms are available to keep automatic check on the following: low oil pressure, high engine temperature, failure of cooling water flow, high bilgewater, engineroom fire, unauthorized entry, explosive vapor. The source of the electric current for operation is the boat storage battery, with a standby dry battery to cover boat battery failure.

The sensor/sender of engine oil pressure and temperature is similar to that used on automobiles. The sensor for the bilge is a float switch that closes its contacts at a preset water level. This

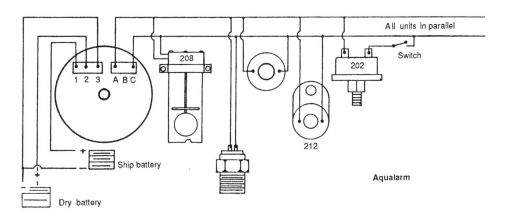

ALARMS—The various sensors available to ensure boat safety are shown in their circuit positions. These sensors (together with the master) will warn of engine temperature, bilge height, oil pressure, etc. *(Courtesy Aqualarm)*

ALTERNATORS

level is slightly higher than the bilge pump operating range and does not interfere.

The vapor detector makes use of the chemical reaction between the explosive or flammable vapor and a rare metal element. The resultant change in resistance is indicated on a meter calibrated in colored zones showing the relative danger of explosion. Audible warning is added. (See also Vapor Alarms.)

State-of-the-art fume detectors no longer restrict their surveillance exclusively to the vapors of gasoline. Today's instruments are also responsive to the tank gases used in cooking and heating and to the highly volatile solvents.

Installation The wiring for these alarms is similar to doorbell wiring and presupposes no experience. The voltage is 12 volts and shockproof. Recommended wire is double-conductor insulated copper No. 18, No. 20, or No. 22. The internal "wiring" of the control panel (when used) is printed circuit.

Maintenance All of the unauthorized-entry and failure-to-function alarms are passive systems and draw no current unless they are activated. The flammable vapor alarm draws a small current as long as it is turned on.

There is no call for maintenance other than checking connections for corrosion and keeping wires out of the bilge and protected. It is advantageous to operate the systems occasionally to make certain they remain at the ready. This is done by momentarily shorting the connections to the normally open switches and opening the circuit to the normally closed switches for an instant. In both cases, the bell or horn should sound. The flammable-vapor detectors have built-in means for testing.

Troubleshooting Troubleshooting is accomplished by tracing the wiring and comparing it with the manufacturer's diagram.

Repair In general, none of the components of these alarm systems is repairable. However, any defective switch is taken out of the circuit easily and can quickly be replaced with a new one of the same type.

Alternators

The alternator has replaced the generator as the engine accessory that supplies the direct electric current to keep the storage battery charged. The superiority of the alternator resides in its ability to deliver more current at lower engine speeds and in its simpler construction that eliminates the commutator with its brushes. The alternator actually is two units within the single housing: the rotating system that generates the current, and the diode combination that rectifies it.

A rotating winding (the rotor) turns at the center of a stationary winding (the stator). A closely controlled current from the battery (see Voltage Regulators) turns the rotor into a multipolar magnet whose lines of magnetic force "cut" the stator and thereby generate an electric current. This generated electricity is a three-phase alternating current (AC) and is unsuitable for battery charging. (The battery current for energizing the rotor reaches it

ALTERNATORS

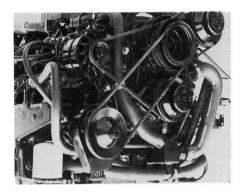

ALTERNATORS—Note the handy-for-service location of the alternator on this popular marine engine. *(Courtesy Mercury Marine)*

via two light-duty brushes and slip rings that are not to be confused with the heavy-duty brushes and commutator of a generator.) Technically, this alternator is said to have a "rotating field."

The alternating current is fed internally to the bank of diodes. A diode is a simple solid-state device that permits electric current to flow in only one direction—by definition, a direct current (DC). The original alternating current thus leaves the alternator as a direct current suitable for battery charging and other purposes (see Diodes).

The amount of current delivered by the alternator depends upon the speed at which it is driven and upon the level to which the rotor is energized by the battery through the voltage regulator—and overall by the condition of the battery charge. The correctly functioning system keeps the battery fully charged without undercharge or overcharge.

The alternator is a rugged unit available for 12-volt DC installations. It contains its own cooling fan within the housing.

Maintenance Maintenance of the alternator is simple in the extreme, because it requires no lubrication. The bearings have been lubricated for life and are inaccessible. Attention should be paid to the condition of the driving belt and to its tightness. Finger pressure at the center of a wide belt span should depress it not more than ½ inch (with the engine stopped, of course). The pivot bolt and the tensioning bolt should be tight. Connecting wires should make clean, bright metal contact. If the battery remains charged during periods of normal usage, the alternator may be considered to be operating normally. A squealing belt during periods of heavy charging is not abnormal and may be overcome with appropriate sprays.

Troubleshooting Troubleshooting an alternator is accomplished with a VOM (see Voltometers). This instrument can check shorts and grounds and continuities of the windings, in addition to identifying good and bad diodes.

Windings must not be "grounded." In other words, the VOM, when on its resistance scale, must indicate infinity when the meter leads are touched to a slip ring and the shaft of the rotor with all other connections removed.

The one-way characteristic of a diode makes possible a simple test with a VOM. With the meter leads on the two terminals of a diode, the meter resistance reading may be high or low. But reversing the leads must give the opposite reading in order for a diode to

15

AMPLIFIER SYMBOLS

be declared good. The same reading in both positions condemns the diode.

Repair The design and construction of the alternator takes it out of the realm of do-it-yourself repair. The usual procedure with an unsatisfactory unit is to exchange it at an automotive electric shop.

The ammeter on the console is the instrument to "read" in determining the condition of an alternator. But careful, commonsense analysis must be used, because there is a possibility for confusion. The observations are made with the engine running at various speeds.

The standard electrical hookup for meter and alternator permits a false zero reading, even while charging is taking place. This occurs when the amount of current being drawn from the battery and the current produced by the alternator are exactly equal. The important caution here is that there should never be a minus condition with engine running—except, possibly, when a heavy-drain item like a big searchlight, for instance, is simultaneously being used.

The average alternator has the ability to put out approximately 30 amperes at 12 volts, the equivalent of 360 watts direct current. Special so-called "truck" models can double this output to supply current for special situations.

Amplifier Symbols

All mental disciplines have their shorthand that imparts nothing to the layman but gives a full story to the initi-

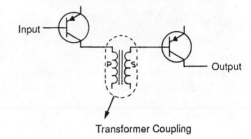

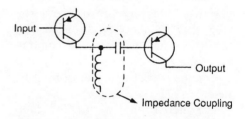

AMPLIFIER SYMBOLS—The symbols for depicting three type of electronic amplifiers are shown. The text explains each.

ated. Medical doctors use far-fetched three-letter abbreviations and compound the mystery with illegible writing. Radio technicians, by contrast, use symbols that are marvels of meaning and are easily understood. Samples of symbols are shown in the accompanying diagrams of transistor amplifiers.

The three elements of a transistor are located within the circles. These elements are the "base" (a bar), the "collector" (a line), and the "emitter" (a line with an arrowhead pointing to the bar for a P transistor and away from the bar for an N transistor). The elements form the input and output terminals of the transistor, as marked.

The type of semiconductor (and its doping) of which the transistor is made determines its classification as P or N (positive or negative) and therefore the polarity of the subsequent battery connection (see Transistors). Connecting to the working battery terminal is "fatal" to a transistor. The diagrams also show three methods of amplifier internal interconnection. Each of the three couplings has its special usage. The difference arises from the contents of the area within the dotted line. The empty area represents direct coupling, for achieving wide frequency response. The inductance and capacitor in the dotted area are impedance coupling (impedance is the alternating-current equivalent of direct-current resistance). Substituting a transformer produces transformer coupling. These three forms of coupling make it possible to adapt the transistor to the impedance requirements of various electronic circuits.

Anchoring

Anchoring takes place either under stress in foul weather, or else as a pleasurable interlude during a cruise. In both situations, the same rules apply because anchoring is both an art and a science, with experience being the best teacher. (See also the next section, Anchors.)

Rule number one is "Know your bottom!" The nature of the bottom in a popular anchorage is usually known by word of mouth. Failing in that, the chart is a reliable source of information. Short abbreviations for what ground cover exists cover the chart and are explained below. The purist may even bring up a sample of the bottom by applying grease to the lead of his lead line (see Lead Lines).

The most accurate measurement of water depth is made with a lead line—but this is an unhandy gadget to use under most conditions. The depth sounder is a good substitute if experience has found it to be accurate. (The distance that the keel extends below the transducer must be subtracted from the reading.)

There seems to be a natural urge among newcomers to throw the anchor forward from the bow. The anchor should *not* be thrown, and, luckily, most anchors are too heavy to permit much throwing. The boat is brought slowly to a dead stop directly over the agreed spot for anchoring, and the anchor is *dropped.* The boat is backed slowly until the desired length of rode (line) has been payed out. The line is snagged to the forward sampson post (or equivalent). A short burst on the throttle, still in reverse, digs the anchor in. A taut line now signals that the anchor is holding.

The foregoing anchoring maneuver is easy to perform with a powerboat. It is much more difficult under sail because of the absence of controlled power. A workable plan is to come to the anchorage with wind abeam and mainsail only. Trimming the mainsheet controls headway to approxi-

ANCHORING

mate the throttle of the powerboat, and the powerboat routine may be followed. The boat drifts with the wind while anchor rode is payed out—and comes to with a snap when the anchor takes hold.

Note that this anchored boat will rule a circular area whose radius is as long as the scope with the anchor as the center. Other nearby anchored boats will have their own circular areas of interference, and there must be no possibility of overlap with a weather change.

Some types of bottoms are Nature's challenge to the anchoring boatman. Dense vegetation licks almost every design of anchor. Loose sand has minimal holding ability. Rocky bottoms often claim anchors for keeps. Abrasive conditions call for chain between anchor and nylon rode.

Setting a muddy anchor on a scrubbed deck is a capital offense, in the opinion of most skippers. Securing the anchor in an awash position during the following run is one easy cleanup method; rinsing the anchor up and down during retrieval is another. Some large boats have a seawater pump at the bow for spraying mud off the anchor.

Maintenance The following cautions are for absent-minded skippers: Make certain the bitter end of the rode is secure. Tie the pin of the anchor shackle with wire. Secure the pin of the stock (where used) with wire.

The above-water source of damage to the rode is the chafing that may take place at the chock that brings the line aboard. The standard remedy is a short length of garden hose. The hose is split lengthwise, placed around the line at the chock, and taped closed with a short tail of tape to keep the hose in place.

Troubleshooting Sometimes an anchor refuses to break out, and getting away becomes more troublesome than the original anchoring. The trick now is to let Nature do the work, if possible, by taking advantage of the boat's buoyancy.

Bring the bow directly over the anchor. Take all slack out of the rode, give an extra heave to bring the bow down, and secure to a cleat or sampson post. Wave motion from wind or traffic, plus movement of persons aboard, should break out the anchor within minutes.

Of course, there are situations when a rocky bottom will defy all efforts except those of a diver. Sadly, the solution then is a sharp knife and a subsequent trip to a marine store.

A handy preventive measure that may help avoid this inconvenience is to rig a "trip line" before anchoring; see Anchors (maintenance section).

The amenities, both social and legal, required of an anchoring skipper depend on the size of his boat and on the nature of the area where he is putting his hook down. Designated anchorages shown on the chart ease the rules. The most important practical consideration is assurance that swinging on its rode does not permit the boat to harm either itself or another vessel.

Vessels less than 65 feet long need not show a light at night nor a ball by day in an anchorage area. (Both light and ball are mandatory for boats anchored in or adjacent to a fairway.)

Anchors

To the landlubber, the anchor is a simple device that holds a boat to the ground when necessary. The sailor knows that anchors and anchoring are, unfortunately, not that simple. There are several styles of anchors, and the correct choice is governed by immediate local conditions. Often the anchor determines the survival of the ship.

The basics of anchoring have not changed over the years, although the design of anchors has. The improvements have one goal: to achieve a construction that will dig itself into the ground most effectively when the anchor is pulled over the bottom. The amount of pull it can resist per pound of weight, when firmly set into the bottom, is a measure of the anchor's effectiveness. Included in this appraisal is the anchor's ability to overcome weeds and other bottom obstacles to its digging.

The original, ancient shape of the anchor is known to almost everyone. From this has evolved a series of modern anchors, with each new style claiming certain advantages in holding ability and digging power. At best, an anchor is a clumsy thing and usually presents a problem in stowage, and this, too, is a determining factor in selecting an anchor for a pleasure boat.

The more popular anchors available today include: the kedge, the Northill, the CQR, the Bruce, and the Danforth. The latter two are the ones generally to be found on pleasure boats. In addition there are two special-purpose anchors: the grapnel, and the mushroom.

The kedge anchor and the Danforth anchor each have a crossbar called the "stock," but the CQR (secure) anchor is stockless. Larger boats equipped with a hawsepipe can stow the CQR and the Danforth there but not the kedge, because its stock interferes. The wide flukes of the Danforth tend to be a disadvantage on grassy bottoms, because they casue the anchor to slide instead of digging. The kedge with its thin arms seems to dig right through thick growths. The CQR is becoming increasingly popular because of its effectiveness on all bottoms.

Danforth anchors are available in three series determined by the grade of steel of which they are manufactured. The standard Danforth is made with basic untreated steel. The next higher quality features chrome molybdenum heat-treated steel and has higher-per-unit holding power. The top-quality and highest-holding-power Danforth is fashioned of premium alloy steel, heat treated for toughness and strength. Hot-dipped galvanizing imparts a protective coating of zinc.

An anchor is in its most effective attitude for digging when its shank is parallel to the bottom. However, this position does not occur when the anchor is being towed by a boat, because then the shank points up at a more or less acute angle. The most common way to overcome this difficulty is to attach a length of heavy chain to the anchor between it and the anchor line ("rode"). The weight of the chain keeps the anchor in its correct digging stance. A plastic-coated chain is cleaner and less damaging to decks; see Anchoring.

ANCHORS

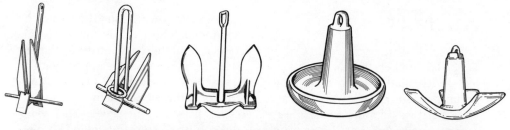

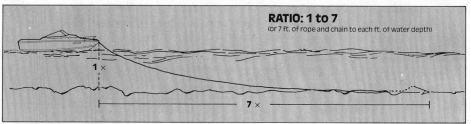

RATIO: 1 to 7
(or 7 ft. of rope and chain to each ft. of water depth)

1. Always use an anchor lead chain to assure optimum penetrating power and stability.
2. The ratio of cable (rope and chain) to water depth should be at least 7 to 1. Penetrating anchors work best when there is plenty of horizontal pull.
3. Most important — be prepared! Different sea bottoms require different anchorages and equipment. Predict conditions ahead of time, and react decisively.

ANCHORS—The drawing illustrates the concept of "ratio" between water depth and rode length for effective holding. Anchor styles vary with manufacturers, with each claiming superior digging in and holding qualities. Shown, l to r, Danforth type, quick release, navy mushroom, river. *(Courtesy ATTWOOD)*

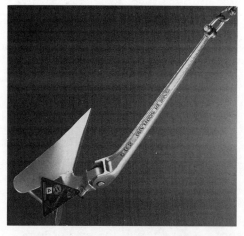

ANCHORS—At A, the Plough anchor, fashioned of cast steel. The manufacturer claims superior release from the bow and quick dig-in. At B, the CQR (secure) constructed of drop-forged steel, claimed to be four times as strong as cast steel. *(Courtesy Jay Stuart Haft CO.)*

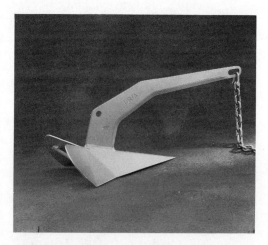

BRUCE ANCHOR—The Bruce Anchor is shown stowed in its special chock. Its makers claim added holding power for this one-piece design, plus ease of digging-in and weighing-out. *(Courtesy Moorings Inc.)*

ANCHORS

The length of rode in relation to the depth of the water is the "scope," and it is obvious that the more rode, the closer the anchor can be to its most effective horizontal digging position. Increasing the scope is always a good answer to a chancy anchoring situation.

The very quality of chain that aids anchoring, its weight, mitigates against it when stowage is considered. An all-chain rode is too heavy for small boats and may even cause difficulties with trim on bigger vessels. It is easily possible for long lengths of chain to cause a bow heaviness that makes a boat sluggish. The answer is to use synthetic line after a length of chain that is just enough for holding the anchor down. (Natural-fiber rope is no longer in use.)

The ideal and almost universal choice for anchor line is nylon. Nylon has elasticity, the ability to stretch and then come back to its original length. This ability brings a bonus when nylon is used for anchoring: It absorbs the hull-wrenching shock when wave action brings the boat up short on its rode. The three-strand twist is the preferred style of rope in use.

Once the necessary anchor weight is decided, the next question is whether or not one person can handle it manually or with a necessary winch (see Winches). The all-rope rode may be belayed to a sampson post or cleat, but the chain section requires a chain stopper and "chain claw" of some form. Whether the anchor is dropped over the bow or through a hawsepipe understandably also changes the method and devices for using it.

The rope and/or chain locker is located directly below the foredeck, at the bow, and access to it is through a deck fitting. Such a fitting has either a cap or a screwplate to prevent the entrance of rain or sea. The prevention of wetness is important because of the locker's tendency to mildew; the nylon does not mind being wet. Usually, the rope being payed through the deck will distribute itself in the locker, although occasionally some human help may be needed to break up a jam. Both anchor and rode should be washed thoroughly by swishing over the side or hosing before anything is fed into the locker. A certain amount of manhandling cannot be avoided.

With an all-nylon rode, the line should end in a spliced-in thimble. A shackle through the thimble then connects rode and anchor. The pin on the shackle should be wired closed with noncorroding wire or with several passes of nylon whipping twine. The soundness of the pin whipping should be checked before each anchoring.

Note that "scope" is a ratio of the length of anchor line deployed to the height of the bow above the bottom.

Maintenance In most rocky-bottom areas, there is always the possibility of the anchor getting jammed and refusing to come up. The protection against this annoyance is rigging a trip line before anchoring. The trip is attached to the crown of the anchor and is slightly longer than the water is deep. At the upper end, the trip line carries a float or a small buoyant cushion so that it may be retrieved.

The bow is brought directly over the trip line so that it may be taken aboard and pulled vertically. If the trip line can be hauled tight and cleated, wave action alone may break the anchor free.

In normal anchoring, the anchor is dropped from the bow at the desired spot. The boat then is slowly backed off by wind or by engine until a "grab" is felt. An extra backward tug then finishes the digging. Unfortunately, this does not always happen as quickly and as smoothly as it can be described.

Leaving an anchorage is somewhat the reverse. The bow is brought directly over the anchor. (This is done by hand signals to the helmsman.) Snugging up the anchor line and cleating it will let wave action break the anchor out.

An anchor down for any length of time in salt water will come up with barnacles almost welded to it. A good wirebrushing is the remedy. Avoid scratching down into the galvanizing.

Antennas

The antenna picks up radio waves for a receiver and forces radio waves into space for a transmitter. To function efficiently, an antenna must have a technical size relationship to the radio waves it is sending and receiving. In other words, the *electrical* length of the antenna must be some multiple of the physical length of the radio wave. (The electrical length and the actual length may differ widely.)

The electrical length of the antenna is adjusted and matched to its destined radio waves by means of "loading coils." These small coils of wire are inserted at calculated points in the antenna construction and cause the radio wave to "think" that it has found a resonant length with which it is compatible. The energy in the wave may now be transferred efficiently to the receiver, or vice versa, from the transmitter. (The loading coils are not visible externally.)

Today's marine radio antennas have boiled down to two shapes: the stainless-steel whip, and the fiberglass pole. Early models included loops and even miles of wire on wooden poles for transatlantic communication. The standard internal antenna for small portable AM radios is a coil of fine wire wound on a powdered-iron core. (See Adcock Antenna, Direction Finder, VHF-FM Radio.)

The operational characteristics of a marine antenna are described by its "band width," its "standing wave ratio" (SWR), and by its "gain." The band width must be wide enough to take the range of frequencies built into the transmitter and receiver. SWR represents an internal loss of power and should be less than 2 (see Standing Wave Ratio). Gain is calculated in decibels (db) and is what the name implies, but there is a drawback: The higher the gain, the narrower the beam, and the greater the chance of a rolling boat missing its target. The terminus of an antenna has a given impedance, in ohms, and this should match the impedance of the coaxial cable for best energy transfer. Antennas on the market are predominantly 3-decibel and 6-decibel, with an occasional 9-decibel.

Antennas are designed to be verti-

ANTENNAS

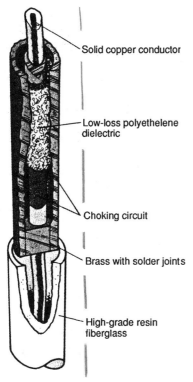

ANTENNAS—Radio antennas are classified as being either Hertz or Marconi, and the difference between the two is shown in the drawings. (The quarter-wave apparently missing in the Marconi is supplied by ground reflection.) The modern whip antenna is a Hertz with the elements "colinear" (in line) and internal. How radio waves are propagated is also shown: (A) Earth wave, (B) line of sight, (C) sky wave. The ionosphere is a reflective shield about the Earth. Atmospheric conditions and frequency determine the mode of travel.

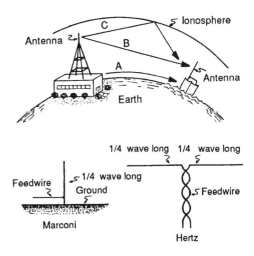

cally or horizontally polarized. This is the position in which they are most effective as receivers and transmitters of radio waves.

Television is now common on pleasure boats, and the antenna makers have been ready. The TV antenna is contained in a compact housing adapted to fastening to the mast. The antenna is omnidirectional, and the original electric motor rotator has been eliminated. Built in with the antenna is a solid-state amplifier to give the TV signals a boost into the connecting cable to the TV. Current for the amplifier travels through the cable also. This TV antenna is claimed to be equally effective for UHF, VHF, and FM.

Installation Antennas should be installed on board where they can have the clearest "vision" all around the compass. It should not be a spot where the whip or pole could provide an inadvertent handhold. Clearance must be available to swing the antenna down to clear bridges. The height of the antenna above the water is a strong factor in communicating range.

ANTENNAS

Maintenance The rod antenna should be wiped down frequently to clear away the salt film that can conduct a high-resistance short. Metal parts should be checked for corrosion.

Directional Antennas

Directional Antennas "aim" at their targets for both reception and transmission without rotary or physical movement. The equivalent for rotational aiming is obtained electronically by sensitive circuits that compare the voltages generated in the various antenna elements.

One form of directionable antenna mounts a vertical rod at each corner of a horizontal square. A suitable shielded cable connects the rods individually to electronic circuits that measure voltage and phase. (Phase is the geometric relationship of one wave to another.) Electronic vectorial addition then reveals the direction in which the antenna is "aimed" for reception or transmission.

An incoming radio wave "cuts" the vertical rods at sufficiently different angles to be electronically recognizable and vectorially usable. The actions for transmission are similar but at higher energy levels. A dial or other indicator relates antenna's azimuth to compass or chart.

Installation Efficient and trustworthy operation demands that the directionable antenna be located where it has a clear all-around "view." There should be no nearby metal to cause confusing reradiation.

Maintenance An occasional wipe to remove salt encrustation (possible short circuit) should meet the requirements.

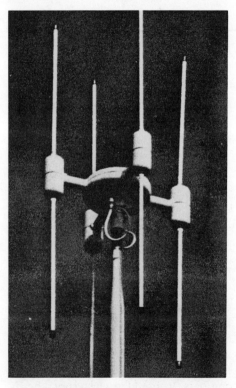

ADCOCK ANTENNAS—The Adcock is a directional antenna that does not require mechanical rotation to function. (The "rotation" is electronic.) Four whips are located at the corners of a square; electronic circuits compare the signal strength in each whip from a given transmitter to determine its azimuth.

Autopilots

As has been emphasized so often, autopilots do not *pilot,* they *steer!* But that alone is blessing enough for a skipper who, otherwise, would need to put in a long trick at the wheel.

The electronic makeup of automatic pilots, or autopilots, runs from simple to very complicated. Fortunately, the

AUTOPILOTS

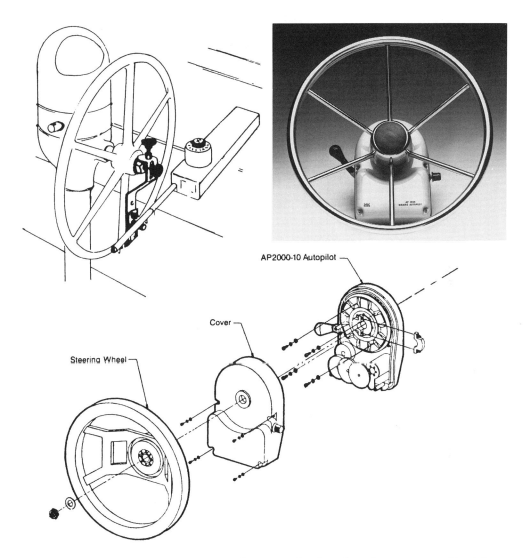

AUTOPILOTS—Three modes of autopilot installation are shown, two for wheel-steered sailboats, one for powerboats. One wheel-steerer turns the wheel directly; the other places an assembly at the wheel hub. *(Courtesy King)* The powerboat unit is cut into the steering system.

complications remain within the black box, and the operation of all commercial autopilots by the skipper is simple in the extreme. "Set the course and keep watch for dangers" is all it amounts to.

The price of autopilots available to the pleasure boater runs from hundreds of dollars to many thousands. The rise in cost of autopilots is in step with the size of boat they are designed to steer. This means that a small sail-

25

AUTOPILOTS

boat may be equipped costwise reasonably, while the owner of a megayacht needs to "dig down deep" to relieve himself of the chore of steering.

Three main components join to form an autopilot: the heading sensor, the power unit, and the control. The sensor maintains the alignment with Earth necessary to hold a course. The power unit does the necessary work of turning the rudder. The control unit accepts the skipper's input of the course to be steered. It maintains this course by constantly comparing it with the north established magnetically or gyroscopically. Many instruments include a feedback circuit that constantly compares the actual movement of the rudder with the angle of deflection requested by the control.

Installation The sensor on the simpler autopilots is a magnetic compass equipped to make electrical contact at the overshoot and undershoot limits of any set course. These contacts start corrective action. (This is known as "hunting.") This compass is as allergic to iron as any other, and consequently is placed in the most deviation-free location on the boat. The next generation of autopilots switched to the fluxgate compass, which has no moving parts (see Fluxgate Compasses). The ultimate sensor is the gyroscope, immune to magnetic problems, and it is standard in the fancy autopilots destined for megayachts (see Gyro Compasses).

The power unit of pleasure-boat autopilots is either hydraulic or electromechanical. The hydraulic power unit is offered in response to the large number of hydraulically steered vessels on the water and coming from the builders. The installation of a hydraulic autopilot is relatively easy; it entails fitting the output of the power unit properly into the existing steering piping according to simple instructions. Of course, the autopilot pump must be able to overcome the boat's steering resistance (see Steering Torque).

The mechanical autopilot power system consists of an electric motor that turns the steering wheel, pulls on a steering cable, or directly turns the rudder. Motors are available for 12-volt, 24-volt, and 32-volt direct (battery) current and, on the large units, for 110-volt and 220-volt alternating current. The control unit governs the motor through relays necessitated by currents too high in amperage for instrument contacts.

Control units run the gamut of designers' ideas. The desired course is fed into the autopilot through a dial, or else the pilot is locked in to the course already being run. Sea conditions are dialed in. (The actual angle the boat will turn in response to a given rudder angle varies with wind, sea, and speed.) The sophisticated autopilot controls obey "orders" from Loran and other navigation systems to produce almost automatic cruising, from one waypoint to the next. It is common for analog or digital course information to be provided at the console and duplicated on the flying bridge.

Autopilots for small sailboats are connected to the steering system directly at the tiller. The power unit on these resembles a cylinder and piston in action, and moves the tiller by pushing against a cockpit seat. One adjustment depends on how far from the rudderpost the autopilot connection to the tiller is made, because this is one of the determinants of the favorable leverage under which the autopilot will function.

All autopilots make provision for "dodging" around dangers that may appear on the course. The dodge is carried out either from a console knob or from a remote activator connected to the autopilot by a long, flexible electric cable. The autopilot remembers the set course during the dodge and returns to it when the skipper releases the dodger (see Self-Steerers).

The more elaborate and more costly autopilots add features that reduce the need for manual attention—for instance, automatic widening of control to allow for weather conditions, off-course alarms, etc.

Maintenance Maintenance is common sense. Many of the controls are claimed waterproof, and that reduces the problem of water seepage into the "works," if the controls are in an exposed position. Check to eliminate any added friction that may increase the load on the autopilot power unit. Note that the sensor compass need not be fully compensated (see Compasses); it is not called upon to read true courses but only *changes* in the course.

Troubleshooting Troubleshooting the autopilot for "out of adjustment" is done by setting a course and using the ship's compass to note disparity. The wake should be straight.

Barometers

A barometer indicates the changes in atmospheric pressure that foretell the weather. However, the optimistic notations on many barometer dials labeled "storm," "fair," etc., are meaningless. Consider a good barometer an extremely sensitive air-pressure gauge.

Barometers are housed in brass cases that often carry steering wheel spokes as a decoration. The manually operable pointer that marks the previous pressure is either brought through the front glass cover or is reached through a hinged door. Experienced skippers set this manual pointer several times a day to coincide with the barometer pointer.

The importance of a barometer reading is not so much the actual pressure but, rather, whether that pressure has fallen or risen. It is the *change* that gives the clue to the weather.

The heart of the barometer is a large, partially evacuated diaphragm, connected through chain and gear with the instrument's pointer. The diaphragm has the atmosphere pressing upon it and moves accordingly. The barometer is "zeroed in" by making its reading coincide with the local weather report, and then noting changes through the day.

Maintenance A barometer requires no maintenance other than occasional wiping or waxing the brass case.

Batteries

Away from the pier, the boatman's electrical helpers derive from his storage battery. The battery either powers the electrical devices directly, or it does so indirectly by starting a generator. Whatever the scheme, the storage battery is the prime source.

BATTERIES

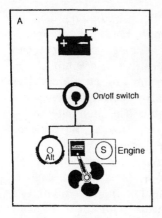
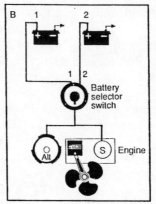
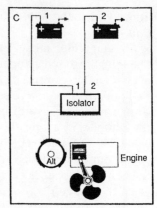
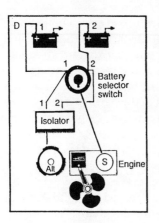
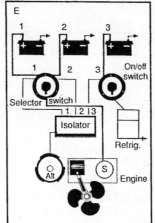
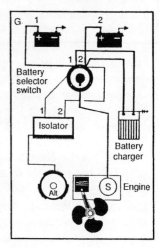
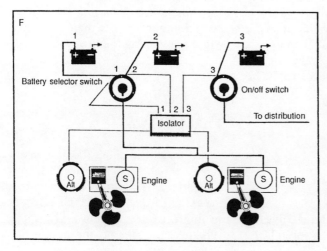

BATTERIES—The "get-home insurance" that comes of having an extra battery aboard is attained by following these wiring diagrams, for single-engine and twin-engine boats *(Courtesy Guest)*

BATTERIES

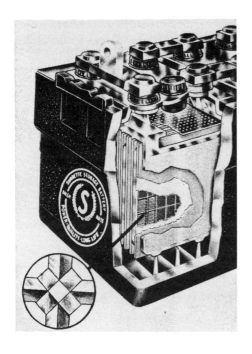

The lead/acid storage battery, the common type, was invented well over a century ago, and its principle of operation remains unchanged, although its construction has been vastly improved. The current storage capacity has been increased, and the bulk has been reduced. The standard terminal voltage is slightly over 2 volts per cell. Thus, the 12-volt boat battery has six cells connected in series (positive to negative to positive, etc.).

Each cell contains two lead electrodes that differ slightly in their chemical composition (the negative electrode is porous lead, the positive electrode is lead dioxide). The electrodes are immersed in dilute sulfuric acid. The lead dioxide of a charged cell becomes lead sulfate on discharge. Charging the cell returns the lead sulfate to its original lead dioxide—and this circle of events may be repeated many times.

The capacity of a storage battery is commercially rated by the amount of current in amperes it can deliver per hour. For instance, 3 amperes per hour for 10 hours would translate to 30 ampere-hours, and the battery is expected to maintain its terminal voltage within 10 percent during the discharge.

Installation The onboard storage battery should be secured against the effects of sea motion. It should be located to give the shortest starting motor cable leads and in an accessible manner that encourages regular testing of its condition. Ventilation is important to dissipate the gas evolved during charge and discharge. (CAUTION: The battery liquid is corrosive, and the battery gas is flammable and explosive.) The battery should have even support to lessen the strain on the plastic battery case. A recently offered addition to the market offers a storage battery that is completely sealed and cannot spill, even when upside down. The electrolyte is in the form of a gel. This battery is claimed to accept freezing without damage.

Maintenance Batteries require simple maintenance, but it must be performed on a continuing, regular, periodic basis. The level of electrolyte liquid must be checked and its hydrometer reading noted. Charging current must be applied whenever this reading falls to an agreed low point. Sulfate and corrosion must be cleared from the terminals whenever they form.

The hydrometer (see Hydrometers) measures the specific gravity of the sulfuric acid solution (a fully charged battery reads around 1280, technically

BEDDING COMPOUNDS (ELASTOMERICS)

Initial Standard Full-Charge Reading at 80°F		State of Charge
1.260	1.280	
1.260	1.280	Fully charged
1.230	1.250	75% charged
1.200	1.220	50% charged
1.170	1.190	25% charged
1.140	1.160	10% charged
1.110	1.130	Discharged

1.280) and is the simplest and most reliable check. A voltmeter has doubtful value unless it is an extremely accurate instrument reading in tenths of a volt.

The table above is for hydrometers with exact scales. The standard temperature is 80 degress Fahrenheit. Add .004 for every 10 degress above standard, and subtract .004 for every 10 degrees below.

Theoretically, the lead/acid storage battery should have distilled water free of all minerals. Actually, manufacturers seem agreed that water good enough to drink is good enough for the battery. (*Never* salt water!) Pitchers specially adapted for battery filling are available and make this chore a quick job. Battery cells have various means of signaling when the correct fill has been reached.

The low battery is charged back to full by connecting a charge (positive to positive and negative to negative) whose direct-current voltage is a volt or two higher than that of the battery. Modern marine chargers shut themselves off automatically at the point of full charge. Without this guardianship, the battery should be checked at intervals during charging. Incidentally, the low-cost home garage automobile charger is not suitable for marine work because it is not isolated for the wet environment.

Magazine advertisements occasionally tout magic liquids and powders that will increase battery effectiveness. These are worthless and could damage the battery. Note also that storage batteries should not be allowed to remain in a discharged condition for any length of time.

Storage batteries are sold with various lengths of warranty, depending on price and, presumably, quality. Replacements are made by trading an old battery plus cash for a new one.

Bedding Compounds (Elastomerics)

The competent boatman fastens nothing to a marine surface without first "bedding it down." Translated, this means that he applies a layer of bedding compound between the surface and the item to be fastened. The purpose is to seal out moisture and fouling organisms; any adhesive strength added becomes a bonus.

Many sealing compounds are available in the marketplace, but only three types are truly suitable for use on boats. Technically, these are polysulfides, polyurethanes, and silicones, and they are sold under various trade names. All three are supplied to the

BEDDING COMPOUNDS (ELASTOMERICS)

user in toothpaste-like consistency that subsequently cures to a synthetic rubber with strong adhesive ability. The cure is a chemical process that, in the case of the polysulfides, requires a catalyst but in the other two is self-contained.

Since the polysulfides are a two-part system, curing time may be controlled over a narrow range by monitoring the percentage of catalyst added. The polyurethanes cure by absorption of moisture and heat and so are dependent upon ambient conditons. This is true also of the silicones. In each case, the curing process first forms a surface skin and then continues through the internal mass. The day after application finds the curing of these sealants at a useful stage, but total chemical cure may not be reached for a week more.

The "rubber" formed by these compounds is sufficiently tough to withstand sanding. This requirement would arise, for instance, when they become the fillers between the strips of a laid wooden deck and must be made flush.

The adhesion of these compounds may be taken for granted and relied upon in all but a few special circumstances. One of these would be their use on woods that may exude oil, such as teak and cedar; here, a special primer must first be applied to the wood.

The three synthetic-rubber compounds are classed together as "elastomerics." One field of maximum usage is the caulking of seams, but this is rapidly diminishing because of the phasing out of wooden boats. In the caulking procedure, a strand of special cotton "rope" is forced into the bottom of the seam as a closure, with the elastomeric then added as a waterproofer flush with the hull.

The "bedding down" mentioned earlier entails laying down a thin layer of elastomeric the size of the base that is to be attached. Tightening the subsequent screws or bolts squeezes out the excess. A quick, careful wipe around the base then leaves a protective fillet.

The elastomerics are expensive compounds, and their high cost often diverts boatmen to cheaper materials such as the caulks sold in supermarkets. Unfortunately, this is a road to disaster, because these bargain "gooks" are unable to combat the marine environment.

The application "technique" for the elastomerics simmers down to putting the stuff exactly where it is wanted and avoiding contact where it is not. (These materials are hard to clean up.) Masking tape is a great helper when lined up carefully with the edge of the seam. Overshoot goes on the tape—and the tape is removed.

The tubes in which the compound is packaged have nozzles that may be used for filling seams, with a putty knife giving the final pressure. Filling a standard caulking gun becomes questionable because of the small quantity (approximately 3 ounces) contained in a tube. A popular catalog lists the availability of elastomerics in clear, white, and brown.

The manufacturer can (and does) make elastomerics that achieve predetermined degrees of fully cured hardness. These various grades do not seem to be in the stocks of marine stores. High-viscosity grades are also made for

BENCH TESTS

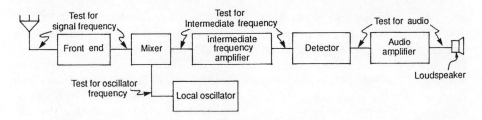

BENCH TEST—How a superheterodyne radio receiver is bench tested, point-to-point, is explained by this diagram. The first point at which a signal is absent borders the trouble. Note changes in frequency.

use on vertical seams where the standard mix would "run." Some yard workers use acetone as a cleanup solvent. (Caution: Acetone is dangerously flammable. This solvent cannot be handled too carefully with respect to fire, lungs, and skin.)

If the work schedule premits a delay, then it is advantageous to choose a hot, muggy day for outdoor work with the elastomerics. High temperature and high humidity cut down curing time for all the compounds. Even the quickest cure is not fast enough to interfere with the average bedding or sealing job.

Typical uses for these elastomeric bedding and sealing compounds are: ports, through-hull fittings, hatches, windows, topside fittings. Another important usage is the stopping of small, annoying leaks at their points of entry. The elasticity of the compounds allows their use even where there is slight "give" between the two surfaces.

Bench Tests

Your radio suddenly goes silent. After tapping it here and tapping it there, you decide it has gone beyond local voodoo magic, and you ship it off to the technicians at the radio repair shop. What strange rites do they perform? The answer is, "None." They use point-to-point testing.

The principle behind point-to-point testing is illustrated by the diagram. A signal, either received or locally generated, is injected into the input of the suspected radio. The presence of this signal or its counterpart is then verified at every successive point down line. An absent signal marks the location of the radio's problem.

The equipment required for point-to-point testing of radio receivers includes a signal generator, and a signal tracer or oscilloscope. The change in the signal as it passes through the various units of the radio circuit must be taken into account. For instance, in the circuit shown, a superheterodyne, the input frequency becomes the intermediate frequency, and then the audio frequency; an oscillator generates a local frequency. (Heterodyning is the mixing of two frequencies to produce a third.)

Bilge Blowers

A bilge blower installation is not only an excellent investment in safety, it is a legal requirement for inboard powerboats. However, there is a caution here: If the blower is to be placed low in the bilge, the motor should be of sparkless construction. (Direct-current [battery-powered] motors have commutators and brushes that may be a source of sparks.)

These are generally centrifugal blowers and differ from fans in that their rotors are "squirrel cages." Input is to the center, with output from the periphery of the housing. The units are rated by the number of cubic feet of air they can move in one minute. An average current requirement for the small 12-volt models is 5 amperes, or 60 watts, with larger-capacity units doubling or tripling this.

Installation When blowers are mounted high in the hold, the pickup of fumes is through flexible hose, 3 or 4 inches in diameter and wire-reinforced to keep it from collapsing under suction.

The additional electrical part needed for a bilge blower installation is a single-pole, single-throw switch of whatever style is desired.

Blowers may also be aboard for passenger comfort (see Ventilation) or as components of air-conditioning units.

Maintenance Some blower motors have provision for oiling; others use oil-impregnated bearings. Note that fan and blower rotors have a tendency to collect dirt. Clamshell fittings or louvers cover the hole where the blower output goes through the hull.

Bilge Pumps

The never-ending struggle to keep the bilges dry revolves around an efficient bilge pump. Since the problem is the same in large boats and small, it is not surprising to find competing manufacturers offering similar pump designs. In general, the actual pump is separate from switches or other accessories. One exception places the pump, a float switch, and a belt-driven impeller into a screened housing that keeps the motor above the water.

The standard construction is a 12-volt direct-current motor, with a shaft-mounted impeller at its lower end, supported vertically in a plastic housing. Restricted openings allow bilgewater to be drawn to the impeller but restrict flotsam that could break it or lock up the pump. Current drain is moderate, considering the volume of water moved.

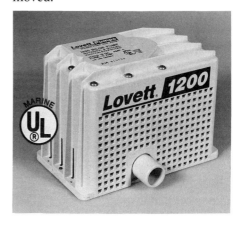

BILGE PUMPS—Most bilge pumps are installed with separate switches to monitor the water level. Shown here is a combination pump and switch in a single housing. *(Courtesy Lovett Pumps)*

BILGE SWITCHES

The bilge pump is controlled either by an automatic switch or manually or by both together (see Bilge Switches). In a properly functioning system, the level of bilgewater is kept below the set point and may be lowered even further with the manual control.

Bilge pumps are sold and priced on the basis of their pumping capacity in gallons per hour. Here there is a caution for the buyer: The rating is made with the pump operating at zero lift—in other words, with the input and output at the same level. This is fine for advertising but of no use in ridding the hull of water. The output must be high enough over the bilge to discharge above the waterline. Unfortunately, this lift usually cuts the pump's actual output approximately in half.

Installation The bilge pump should be installed in the hull at the lowest point of the bilge. Open limber holes should provide easy bilge drainage to this point. (These pumps are the centrifugal type that develop little intake suction and therefore cannot be located above the bilge level.) The pumps come with two long wire leads, and all connections should be made well above any possible bilgewater level.

Recently, the industry changed its electric motor from wire-wound field coils to permanent magnet fields. This makes polarity of installation important. The coded positive wire *must* be hooked up to the positive line from the battery (through switches, of course). Reversal of polarity will cause these permanent magnet pumps to run backwards.

From the standpoint of possible dangerous sparking in the bilges of gasoline-powered boats, these bilge pumps are reasonably safe. The commutator brushes are inside a tightly closed steel shell.

Maintenance The motors of these pumps are lubricated for life at the factory, and there is no provision for maintenance oiling in the field. Observation and removal of any debris impeding water flow is the extent of required attention.

Troubleshooting Troubleshooting a recalcitrant pump is simple in the extreme: Check to assure that the impeller shaft is free and not frozen. Connect the pump to a 12-volt battery. If it runs at high speed, the unit is okay. If it does not run, replace it. There is no repair.

Bilge pumps require onboard direct-current power in the form of a charged storage battery. Many sailboats do not carry this but are equally in need of a bilge pump. For these vessels there are hand-operated bilge pumps.

These hand pumps generally are of the diaphragm construction. They are built with large flapper valves that don't mind sucking up an occasional cigarette butt. One model fastens under the cockpit sole and accepts its operating handle through a flush deck plate. Inserting the handle and rocking it back and forth does the pumping. Flexible input hose picks up bilgewater; flexible output hose discharges overboard.

Bilge Switches

Many small boats come equipped with a bilge pump connected to a single-

BINOCULARS

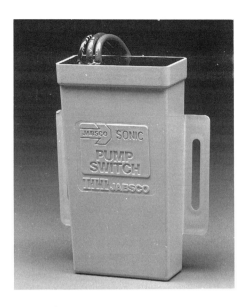

BILGE SWITCHES—This latest entry into the bilge pump switch field makes use of ultrasonic waves to sense water height. Timed relays ensure that pumping is completed. *(Courtesy ITT Jabsco)*

pole, single-throw switch on the console. However, relying on the skipper's memory to keep the bilge safe is not the best procedure. An automatic switch that keeps watch day and night is better, and it enhances the feeling of security.

Bilge switches come in a variety of shapes, sizes, and types, and some are incorporated into a unit with the pump. The basic element of the automatic types is a so-called mercury switch that consists of two contacts and a globule of mercury sealed into a glass tube. Tilting the tube causes the mercury to engulf the contacts and turns the current on. (Theses switches are obviously vapor-proof.) A float arrangement tilts the tube when the preset bilge level is reached. Switches of this design are fastened to the hull and are constantly submerged.

The destructive power of seawater being what it is, designers have tried various schemes to keep the bilge switch high and dry. One method causes the rising bilgewater to compress the air in a diaphragm, through tubing, and this closes a switch. Another idea places two contacts above the bilge at a height that will be short circuited when the water rises. The latest wrinkle on the scene projects supersonic waves at the bilge surface and functions off the reflection.

All good switches have an interval between "on" and "off." They will turn on at the preset maximum water height and turn off at a much lower acceptable level. This feature prevents continuous on/off annoyance.

Installation All connections should be made well above possible maximum bilge height. Tape does *not* prevent the entry of water and subsequent failure by corrosion.

Maintenance Part of maintenance is to move the float up and down manually to check on proper response from the pump.

Binoculars

Binoculars increase the skipper's "seeing power." They bring him as many times closer to the subject as the magnification number of the glasses. Thus, 7 × 50 binoculars bring the view seven times closer than the naked eye can see it. (Fifty is the diameter, in millimeters, of the object lens.) Incidentally, 7 × 50 is the favored spec for boating binoculars. The larger the object lens, the better for night viewing, because more light enters.

Two types of binoculars are manufactured: the "straight-through," with the long barrels, and those with internal prisms and short barrels. The prisms bend the light beams back and forth and reduce the necessary length. Boating binoculars are predominantly of the prism type.

The internal structure of binoculars consist of a series of lenses and prisms closely fitted to each other and cemented together with Canadian balsam. This adhesive is used because its light-transmitting characteristics are nearly identical with those of glass.

Binoculars vary in price from very moderate to extremely expensive. By and large, "you get what you pay for." The expensive units are more accurately constructed and give brighter images because they waste less of the light passing through.

Binoculars are available with internal magnetic compasses whose readings are superimposed on the scene being viewed. This permits a simultaneous bearing to be obtained. Some binoculars are claimed waterproof to a depth of many feet, but testing the veracity of the claim is not advised.

Binoculars are either center focus, wherein a central thumb wheel focuses both barrels together, or individual focus. The center focus adds focusing on one barrel to enable compensation for difference in the eyes. Specifications for binoculars include the width of the field of view at 1,000 yards, exit pupil in millimeters, whether lenses are coated, relative brightness, protection against moisture. Some binoculars are filled with nitrogen gas to prevent fogging and to guard against the influx of water. Soft rubber eye caps are a great help in comfortable binocular use.

Maintenance Despite the manufacturer's claims of sturdiness, binoculars should be treated gently. Most important, the strap should be around the user's neck at all times—just in case. The habitual use of lens caps, front and back, is an excellent practice.

Blocks

A block is a unit of tackle consisting of two sides, called "cheeks," between which is fitted a rotating, wheel, or "sheave." The sheave is grooved for the passage of a line. Blocks are used to increase the ratio of pulling force or to change its directions. Two blocks connected by the line "reeved" (threaded) through them are called a "block and fall." One common use for a block and fall is on a davit for handling dinghies and anchors.

The line must be reeved (threaded) through standard blocks. "Snatch blocks," which open, make reeving unnecessary.

Present-day blocks have cheeks made of plastic, aluminum, steel, or titanium.

All blocks should be rinsed free of salt and dirt periodically and lubricated.

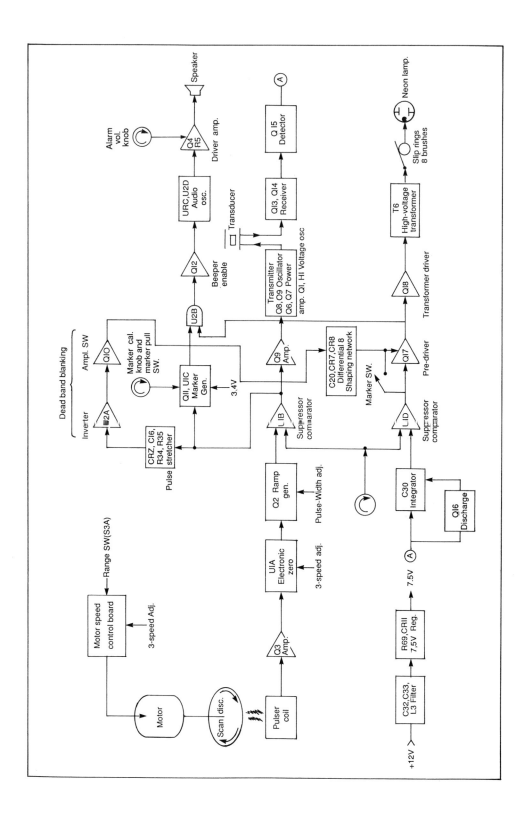

BLOCK DIAGRAMS

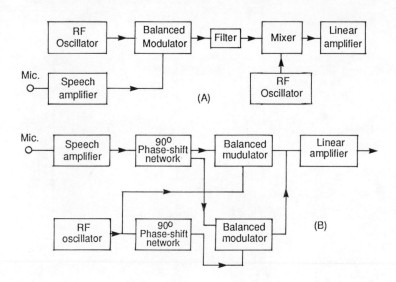

BLOCK DIAGRAMS—The complex block diagram shows each step in the operation of a depthsounder. (Courtesy Lowrance Electronics) The other block diagram shows two methods of achieving single-sideband operation, (A) by *filtering* out the carrier and one sideband and (B) by *balancing* out the unwanted carrier and sideband. *(Courtesy American Radio Relay League)*

Block Diagrams

Electronics manufacturers usually explain their circuits by including block diagrams in their owner's manuals. The layman can understand these diagrams and can comprehend what is taking place without technical expertise. Such understanding often leads to more effective use of the equipment and a more helpful report if failure occurs.

The makeup of a block diagram is simplicity in the extreme. Plain rectangles take the place of the exact symbols in an engineering drawing. The rectangles each contain a plain-English statement of what occurs at that point in the circuit under normal operation. Triangles indicating amplifiers may be included under modern conventions. Circuit tracing in the event of trouble becomes the repetitive asking of the same question: What should be happening at this rectangle that is not taking place?

Actual block diagrams are shown to illustrate their adaptability to a simple circuit and to a complex one. Tracing is carried on serially from input to output.

Bow Thrusters

A boat moving forward steers like an automobile going backward. To turn

BOW THRUSTERS

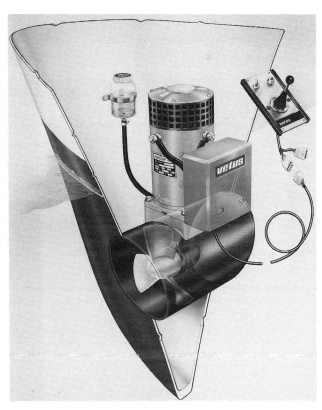

BOW THRUSTER—This bow thruster is installed far forward, below the waterline, with its "tunnel" connecting an opening in the port bow with a companion opening in the starboard bow. The propeller throws water in either direction for right or left thrust. The control is by switch from the bridge. *(Courtesy Vetus)*

the bow to the left, the stern must be pushed to the right. The bow has no steering ability of its own (unless a bow thruster is provided), and the opposite movements of bow and stern take place about a center located approximately at the mid-length of the hull.

The bow thruster "steers" the bow by pushing against one side of the hull or the other. Thus, if the boat is to be steered to the left, the rudder would push the stern to the right and the bow thruster would move the bow to the left, thereby creating a controlled turn. Steering the boat to the right would mean a reversal of the directive forces. The effect now mirrors a car whose front and back axles both steer. The bow thruster gives the helmsman close control in tight spots and in strong wind.

Bow thrusters are of two styles. One kind has a tunnel through the hull crossways at the forefoot of the bow. In the tunnel is a power-driven reversible propeller controlled from the helm. The prop ingests water from one side and squirts it out at the other, creating a push. The steersman adds as much of this push as needed to make a desired turn; he does this with a push-button or joystick controller. The bow thruster need be active for perhaps only a minute at a time.

The other style of bow thruster substitutes a high-powered pump and two

BOWDEN WIRES

nozzles for the tunnel and propeller. A nozzle is on each side, near the forefoot, and a remote-controlled valve selects which is to eject. (The nozzle on the right pushes the bow to the left.) The pump sucks its water via a through-hull fitting. Both thrusters use electric motors.

Note that neither system "pushes against the water." Both bow thrusters are *reaction* devices in which every action causes an equal and opposite reaction, in accordance with the laws of physics. The thruster throws a given mass of water, and the reactive force throws the thruster back—and the hull with it.

The ability of bow thrusters is rated in "pound-feet." (A "pound-foot" is a unit of torque or twisting force; see illustration and Steering Torque.) Thruster makers have approximate figures for the pound-foot requirements of various vessels. Voltage requirements for the motors include 12 volts, 24 volts, and commercial voltages.

Installation Some skippers may quake at the thought of two large holes for the tunnel cut into the hull. Vibration and the working of the hull underway could seem like an invitation to leakage, although on metal hulls the tunnel could be welded in. The advantage of the pump system is that only holes for through-hull fittings need be drilled. Of course, both installations require haulout. Installing bow thrusters requires the know-how of a first-class boatyard.

Maintenance Maintenance comprises motor lubrication and keeping the propeller clear of fouling. Cathodic protection may be needed. Shaft seals should be inspected. A shear pin between shaft and propeller protects the unit in case of prop blockage. (A shear pin on a shaft is like a fuse in an electrical circuit: Each "lets go" by sacrificing itself and disconnects before the acting forces can cause damage.) The low-voltage models draw current like a starter, and connections must be tight and free of corrosion.

Bowden Wires

A Bowden wire forms the basic unit of many small-boat steering and engine controls. It consists of a wire inside a flexible tubing. A knob at one end of the wire allows linear pulls and pushes to be transmitted to the other end to perform various types of control. In earlier automobile days, a Bowden wire connected the dashboard with the engine choke.

The Bowden wire is able to deliver pushes as well as pulls because the central wire is closely confined by the tubing or casing. The tubing may be bent to reasonable radii in its run from console to engine or rudder or whatever.

Maintenance Light lubrication of the central wire is advised—not so much to prevent wear (the use of a Bowden is generally intermittent) as to provide ease of operation.

Breaker Points

Gasoline engines older than of recent manufacture depend upon breaker

CAPACITORS

points for their ignition. Modern gas engines time their sparks with magnetic pickups that do not wear down from use, as breaker points do.

Breaker points make and break contact in response to a cam on the distributor shaft that synchronizes the action with the firing requirements of the cylinders. The resultant sparks at the spark plugs take place when a piston is in the desired nearly top dead center (TDC) position.

Breaker points are formed from the toughest alloys, including metals such as tungsten. The ideal contact surfaces for a pair are one flat and the other rounded. The harmful spark that would occur at the breaking of contact is absorbed by a shunt capacitor that is a crucial item in the ignition circuit.

Setting the gap between breaker points is part of the ignition timing process. Standard gaps vary between .010 and .025 inch and are stated in the owner's manual.

The higher the dielectric constant of the dielectric used, the greater the capacitance of the capacitor. (Courtesy ARRL Handbook)

Dielectric Constants and Breakdown Voltages

Material	Dielectric Constant*	Puncture Voltage**
Air	1.0	
Alsimag 196	5.7	240
Bakelite	4.4–5.4	300
Bakelite, mica-filled	4.7	325–375
Cellulose acetate	3.3–3.9	250–600
Fiber	5–7.5	150–180
Formica	4.6–4.9	450
Glass, window	7.6–8	200–250
Glass, Pyrex	4.8	335
Mica, ruby	5.4	3800–5600
Mycalex	7.4	250
Paper, Royalgrey	3.0	200
Plexiglass	2.8	990
Polyethylene	2.3	1200
Polystyrene	2.6	500–700
Porcelain	5.1–5.9	40–100
Quartz, fuxed	3.8	1000
Steatite, low-loss	5.8	150–315
Teflon	2.1	1000–2000

*At 1 megahertz ** In volts per mil (0.001 inch)

Capacitors

A capacitor truly stores electricity as such, in contrast to a storage battery that stores electricity in the form of chemical energy. (In pre-electronics days, capacitors were called "condensers.")

It is unusual to find an electronic circuit without capacitors. In appearance, capacitors are small cylinders, perhaps 1 inch long and ¼ inch in diameter, with two wire connections extruding. The cylinders are marked, digitally or by color code, with capacity in microfarads and permitted voltage. (Excess voltage causes failure by breakdown.) Capacitors have a smoothing and tuning action on an electronic circuit.

Internally, the capacitor consists of two strips of metal foil separated by a strip of insulating paper, the whole rolled up tightly and sealed. When an electric charge is applied, a field of

CARBURETORS

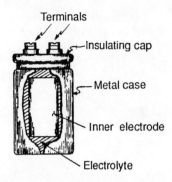

CAPACITORS—The two kinds of capacitors found in electronic equipment are the dry, fixed type (dielectric is paper or film) and the wet electrolytic type (dielectric is oxide formed by the electrolyte). The electrolytic capacitor may be identified by the high capacitance and by the aluminum outer container. The high capacity derives from the thinness of the oxide film dielectric. The life of an electrolytic is shorter than the almost infinite life of a paper capacitor.

stress develops equivalent to the voltage, and this is the storage effect. Shorting the two wires dissipates the charge with a spark.

Large capacitors, like those on motors, should be handled warily. When fully charged at high voltage, they are capable of lethal shock.

Repair The vulnerable part of a capacitor is the dielectric (the insulator). Higher-than-rated voltage causes this dielectric to be punctured, rendering the capacitor useless and not repairable.

Carburetors

The carburetor continuously mixes air and gasoline while the engine is running, and it maintains a predetermined ratio range of the two fluids. The resulting mixture meets the normal flammability requirements of the engine. The carburetor mechanism also provides mixture enrichment for cold starting and "shots" of straight gasoline for acceleration.

Carburetors are classified by their number of main air passages, or "throats." The simplest carburetor has one throat, the most complicated has four throats, and this progression

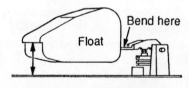

1 Float level adjustment

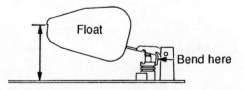

2 Float drop adjustment

CARBURETORS—These drawings show the general principles of adjusting a carburetor float to maintain the desired height of fuel in the bowl. (1) is the adjustment bend for float level; (2) is the bend for float drop. Various makes and models may vary in detail from these drawings but will be sufficiently similar for recognition.

CARBURETORS

would match the increasing size of the engine for which the unit is intended.

The carburetor functions by reducing its internal air pressure below atmospheric. It does this with an "egg-timer"-shaped tube in its throat called a "venturi." The venturi follows the Bernoulli law that the higher the velocity, the lower the pressure. The air sucked in by the downward travel of the engine pistons travels through the venturi at high velocity, and the resulting low pressure causes gasoline to flow in from the carburetor jets and mix with the air. The jets are metered for running speeds, and an adjustable jet regulates the fuel for idling.

So-called "metering rods" in many carburetors automatically adjust fuel flow according to engine load as reflected by changes in manifold vacuum. These are tapered rods whose full diameter closes off the hole in which they move up and down. As the rod is withdrawn to the taper, more of the hole is left open for fuel passage.

Two valves, called "butterfly valves," are under manual control. One is the throttle, and it controls engine speed. It does this by varying the air-flow opening to the throat. The other is the so-called "choke" that enriches the fuel mixture for cold starting by reducing the proportion of air. This choke feature is now automatic on most carburetors and depends upon a thermal spring responsive to engine temperature.

Gasoline reaches the carburetor through the action of a fuel pump situated in the tubing from the fuel tank. The fuel enters the carburetor and is maintained in the bowl at a predetermined level by a float and needle valve mechanism (see Fuel Pumps). The jets connect with and draw upon this reservoir.

Sudden opening of the throttle, as in a demand for greater speed, would stall the engine if no fuel enrichment were provided. For this reason, an accelerating pump is found on every standard carburetor. This device is truly a little pump with a miniature piston in a cylinder connnecting with the bowl. Piston movement is under lever and spring control and makes a downward, pumping stroke upon initial throttle opening. The result is a squirt of gasoline into the carburetor throat. The piston moves only when the throttle does; it is not responsive to steady speed.

The running jets have finely calibrated holes measuring in the few thousands of one inch. Obviously, they could become clogged by dirt or foreign matter. The fuel filter at the input to the carburetor is there to avert such a disaster. This in-line filter is made with extra-fine metal screen and is packed closely with fibrous material; it will remove matter down to micron size.

Marine carburetors, by law, must have a flame arrestor encasing the throat opening. This is a great safety feature because flames cannot travel through the arrestor screen (same principle as the Davy miners' lamp).

Maintenance Maintenance of the carburetor divides into cleaning and observing. The flame arrestor is removed and washed with gasoline (careful!), then air dried. Water-and-soap solutions should not be used, because enough moisture may stay in the screen by capillarity to cause trouble. While the arrestor is off is a good time

CARBURETORS

to check the accelerating pump. Quick opening of the throttle should squirt an easily visible stream of gasoline. Drops of oil on throttle plate and choke plate bearings are advisable. After exposing the float, you can adjust the fuel level in the bowl by bending the float arm. The fuel filter at the input to the carburetor should be checked for unobstructed flow.

Some installations consist of two carburetors working together. It is essential that these two be perfectly synchronized. Synchronization is achieved visually be observing the positions of the two butterfly fuel valves. Any movement of the speed control, such as the throttle, should place the two butterfly disks into identical angles and closures. Threaded actuators allow adjustment. The same reasoning and action apply to the choke plates.

For greater ease in understanding its operation, the carburetor may be divided mentally into the acceleration system, the running-speed system, the choke system, and the idling-speed system.

Troubleshooting The logic here is that the carburetor must have air and gasoline in order to supply a flammable charge to the engine. A dirty flame arrestor could obstruct air; a clogged fuel filter could obstruct gas.

The engine does not run or runs raggedly: Check for the presence of gasoline in the bowl by depressing the accelerating pump and observing the squirt. Check the position of the choke plate with reference to engine temperature (open for warm, closed for cold).

The engine idles rough: Set the idle adjustment screw halfway between too rich (engine slows) and too lean (engine misses). Check the fast-idle cam that automatically sets a higher idling speed to hasten the warm-up. Moving the throttle should disengage the fast idle. Unwanted air (loose or defective gaskets, open vacuum hoses) is a major cause of carburetor malfunctioning, and careful inspection pays off when troubleshooting.

Repair Carburetors are intricately assembled mechanisms, and working on them requires skilled fingers. Repair kits are available for most models and contain the parts most likely to need replacement, plus full directions. It can be a do-it-yourself jog—though a tedious one. The other option is the comparatively easy one of loosening and removing four bolts and unhooking the controls, then making an exchange for a "rebuilt" at a carburetor shop.

Some cautions apply, regardless of carburetor make and model: When two carburetors are standard equipment, both throttle plates are synchronized to control speed, but the choke of only one carb is active in the choking procedure. An adjustment made with the aid of a threaded rod on one model may be made on a competing model by simply bending a linkage.

The plates of the throttle valve and of the choke valve are screwed to their shafts after assembly and may present a removal problem if worn shaft holes make repair necessary. (Worn bearing surface and excessive shaft clearance allow the entry of unwanted air that affects fuel mixture.)

The holes in carburetor jets are drilled to calibrations of fractions of one-thousandth of one inch and need careful handling. Jets should be cleared only with solvent and compressed air—and not with stiff wires or needle drills.

Cavitation

Cavitation is a destructive situation that many high-speed propellers may be heir to. The onset of cavitation is heralded by a distinctive noise and by a sudden speed-up of the engine. Aside from the annoyance, cavitation has the ability to damage the propeller.

At some unique critical combination of positive and negative pressures on the two sides of a high-speed prop, a film of air replaces the contact with the water. The propeller dumps its load, and the engine momentarily tries to run away. The propeller is said to be "cavitating."

Supersonic forces are let loose during the cavitation, and these can damage even a sturdy metal prop. Difficult as it may be to believe, pellets of water now strike the surface of the propeller with sufficient force to make indented pock marks. Cavitation can ruin a propeller if allowed to continue.

High-speed props positioned close to the water's surface are more likely to cavitate. Outboard motors take this into account by providing a "cavitation plate" over the propeller to reduce air ingestion.

Some hull designs "drag" air to the prop region, and this may induce cavitation if other factors are favorable.

Chargers

The primary source of electric current on a pleasure boat is a storage battery. Storage batteries need intermittent recharging to replace the current used. Hence, a battery charger is an almost universal accessory on boats, although

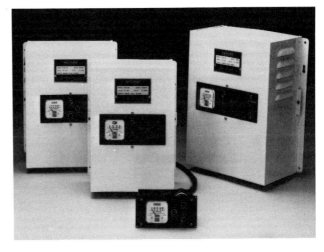

CHARGERS—These battery chargers turn themselves on and off as the batteries require to remain "topped." Internal construction of these chargers insulates ship from shore. Harmful "trickle charge" has been abandoned. *(Courtesy Sentry)*

some small craft make do with the current from the alternator (see Alternators, Batteries).

A battery charger rectifies the pier alternating voltage to direct, the only form the battery will accept. The voltage is reduced to slightly more than battery level, and automatic control is exerted. To accomplish these functions, the charger cabinet contains a transformer, a rectifier, an electronic control circuit, a meter, and switches. Fuses or breakers protect the entire installation of charger and battery.

The control constantly monitors the battery charge level and keeps it optimum by turning the charger on and off as required. An important feature of a good, safe charger is electrical isolation between pier and battery bank.

Charger cabinets allow operation either free-standing or hanging from a bulkhead. The charger is either "on" or "off"; the old idea of "trickle charging" has been abandoned. Popular charger sizes are: 10 amps, 20 amps, 40 amps, and 60 amps. Cabinets are treated to withstand the marine environment.

Maintenance Dust is an enemy of chargers because it clogs louvers and interferes with cooling (most chargers are gravity cooled without fans). Chargers are connected to batteries positive to positive (usually red) and negative to negative (usually black). Chargers in service should not get warmer than "comfortable to the touch." The ammeter indicates the amount of current going into the battery (see Volt and Ampere Meters).

Repair Generally a dead charger is dead because its diodes have failed. It may be financially viable to replace diodes.

Chocks

Chocks are guides that direct a line to a cleat, to a winch, or to other destinations. The chock may be a separate metal fitting attached to the structure of the boat, or a chock may simply be a large hole in the bulwark. The individual chock may be open or closed. The open chock allows line to be set in, while the closed chock requires lines to be run ("reeved") through. (The need to reeve may interfere with quick action.)

The two short horns of an open chock may overlap at an angle and be a short distance apart. This scheme produces an open chock with the continuous control of the line that a closed chock exerts. The favorite metal for chocks is bronze.

All surfaces of the chock that come in contact with the line must be highly polished. Any roughness causes continuous abrasion when the boat "works." One way to prevent line damage is to use split garden hose pieces over the line where it goes through the chock. Fastening a chock in place with only wood screws or sheet-metal screws is not enough, and is not safe (see Cleats).

Circuit Breakers

A circuit breaker, as its name implies, is a simple protective device that breaks the flow of electrical current when an overload occurs. It functions instantly when its set point is reached and thereby prevents damage and possible fire. Circuit breakers are available for a wide list of maximum currents (amperes) and in models for direct current and for alternating current.

Internally, circuit breakers work either magnetically or thermally. The magnetic type has an electromagnet through which the current to the load flows and creates a magnetic field. The more current, the stronger this field. At slightly above the current for which the circuit breaker is calibrated, the magnetism becomes strong enough to trip a switch and open the circuit. The circuit may be reset only manually.

The thermal type of circuit breaker relies on the heating effect of an electric current. The current to the load passes through a heating coil. At the set point, the temperature is high enough to deflect a bimetallic element and open a switch. In another form of thermal circuit braker, the high temperature melts solder and allows a spring to open the switch. In both types, a few minutes, cool-down after opening allows manual resetting.

The type of load to be protected must be considered in choosing a circuit breaker. A motor, for instance, may double its current when starting, whereas a light bulb does not exceed its rating. Thus, the motor needs a slow-acting breaker to permit it to start without instant shutdown.

Installation An overall circuit breaker that shuts everything down is a good idea. The recommended mounting for circuit breakers is all on an adequate panel, with each breaker clearly marked with the circuit it protects. The installation should be accessible and protected from moisture. If lighting can be added to the panel, it is recommended.

Maintenance Connections should be kept clear of corrosion.

Cleats

Cleats are hardware items attached to the boat structure to which lines may be fastened (the sailor says "belayed"). Cleats may be one solid pice of plastic, wood, or metal, or they may be of a design containing movable members that jam the line. Cleats are available in many sizes to suit the load and the boat.

The typical, standard cleat has a base and a rising central neck that supports a protruding horn extending outward on two sides. The neck is high enough to allow a line to be taken around it. Screws going down through the base attach the cleat to the deck or other structure. The whole cleat is polished smooth to avoid damage to the line under strain.

The cleat with movable jaws is found on sailboats where it controls the sheets. The pull on the sheets causes the jaws to close upon the line and secure it tightly. The desirable feature is instant holding and instant release as required.

Cleats of hardwood, especially loved by tradition-conscious sailors, and cleats of plastic, are not as widely used as cleats of metal. The metals in current use are low-cost alloy, stainless steel, and bronze—with the latter preferred.

Installation The most important features about a cleat is how it is fastened to the boat. Simple attachment

COMPASSES

with wood screws or sheet-metal screws is *never* sufficient! The recommended fastening is a bronze bolt with nut and washers. (The bolt may be a carriage bolt style that has a less obstructed head.)

The details of setting the cleat in place start with the drilling of through-holes for the carriage bolts. Bedding compound is spread over the area to be covered by the cleat base, with some going into the bolt spaces (see Bedding Compounds). On the inside below, a properly drilled backing plate covered with bedding compound is slipped over the bolts and tightened in place with nuts and washers. The metals chosen for the bolts and the cleat should be the same. Excess compound is wiped away by running the finger around the edges of the base and the plate to form rounded fillets.

Compasses

"The compass card stands still, and the boat turns around it." That statement, fresh in mind, is the key to understanding the marine magnetic compass. That simple explanation puts the novice at ease during his early attempts to steer in response to compass information.

How fortunate that the Earth is a huge magnet! The resultant surrounding magnetic field affects compasses everywhere and causes them to indicate approximate north. The indication is not *true* north because the magnetic field does not line up with the Earth's geographic poles.

Sections of the magnetic field are further distorted by differences in the magnetic permeability of the Earth, and these are called a "variation" and are shown as lines on a chart. Variation is beyond human correction. Finally, there is a further distortion due to magnetic items aboard; this is "deviation" and is correctible within the compass.

The modern marine compass is essentially a floating magnet with a 360-degree dial attached. The quality of the compass is determined by how quickly the dial aligns itself with north and how faithfully it remains in that alignment despite the motions of the boat.

Most marine compasses are covered by a geometrically true dome of high optical quality that, together with the contained liquid, magnifies the dial. The liquid is a refined oil of low viscosity. (So much for those novelized sailors who got drunk on compass alcohol!) The floating dial is a clever way to dampen motion and to take weight off the jeweled pivot. The assembly is fully gimbaled.

The liquid is contained in the shape of a ball, so that rapid changes in position of the compass during rolls and yaws cause no waves to upset the dial. An expansion chamber leaves no room for air bubbles. A damping system eliminates sudden jerks in dial movement.

The heart of the compass is the directive magnet(s) under the dial. The magnets are of Swedish iron, magnetized, then aged to stablize their magnetic intensity over a period of time.

Dials are calibrated in degrees (no longer in points), with graduations as close as 1 degree for a large compass

COMPASSES

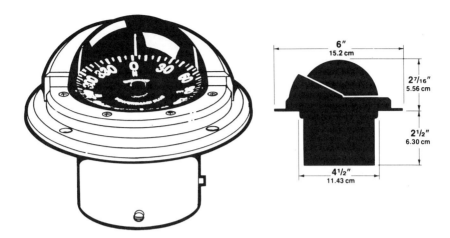

COMPASSES—This popular marine compass has its compensators in the base. One for north/south, one for east/west. *(Courtesy E. S. Ritchie & Sons)*

and 5 degrees, 10 degrees, or other spacings for smaller instruments. Visibility at the compass location should determine the graduations chosen. Most compasses provide a facility for night illumination with red light.

Compensating a compass for onboard deviation used to be done with magnets placed in the area around the compass. The modern marine compass carries its compensators in its base, where they are under the control of a nonmagnetic key. Two keyways are provided, one for north–south, the other for east–west. When each keyway has been turned to a position that has no effect on the dial, the compass *is said to be* "zeroed in" *and ready* for compensation.

Installation Two vital considerations for location of the compass aboard: (1) The lubber line fore-and-aft through the center of the dial must be directly over the keel line or, if to one side, then parallel to it. (2) There must be no magnetic objects within a minimum of 2 feet from the compass in any direction. The mounting surface should be either horizontal or vertical, or corrected to be so.

Maintenance The compass should be wiped clean and waxed regularly, with care taken not to scratch the plastic dome. Magnetic interference should be checked by moving suspected objects and turning electrical circuits on and off while observing the dial for undesired movement. (This becomes especially important after a nearby lightning strike.)

Troubleshooting Compensation of the compass may be checked as follows, with all equipment in seagoing condition:

On a local chart, choose markers or landmarks as the ends of two courses, one running north–south, and the other running east–west. Note the two magnetic bearings from the chart. Run the northerly course, and correct the compass with the nonmagnetic key bearing to agree with the chart. Return

CONTROL CABLES

southerly, and correct to half the error.

Run the east–west course, and correct the compass bearing with the non-magnetic key to agree with the magnetic bearing of the chart. Return on the course, and correct to one-half the error.

Sailboats running these compensation courses should hold heeling to a minimum to avoid the injection of heeling error. (This is a good time to make a deviation table by running courses every 30 degrees and noting the results.)

Repair A leak of fluid or a failure of the expansion chamber will show up as air bubbles. Such damage is easily repairable at the factory.

The only part of a well-kept compass that may wear out is the red-colored light bulb. Incidentally, a rheostat (dimmer) in this circuit is desirable.

CONTROLS—These controls for engine and steering make use of a steel cable within a flexible housing to transmit pushes and pulls. Shown are a twin-engine setup and an explanatory view of cable construction. (Technically, these are Bowden wires.) *(Courtesy Morse Controls)*

Control Cables

Flexible push-pull cable has moved the outboard helmsman forward from the transom to a center console or to the bow. The forward end of the cable terminates in a unit that translates steering-wheel rotation into a push or a pull. The after end of the cable moves the outboard(s) accordingly. A sister cable transmits the movement of the control lever to the gearshift and to the throttle.

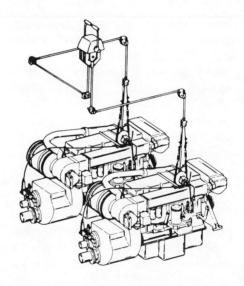

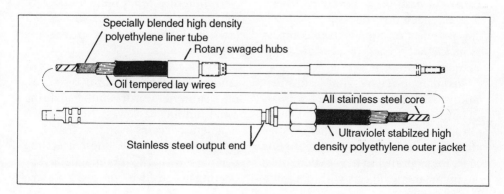

A flexible tube is formed by an arrangement of steel wires and is covered by a plastic jacket. Within this tube, a central core of steel wires slides back and forth as required. Proper end fittings connect the core to whatever job is needed to be done. The cable is a greatly beefed-up and improved version of the "Bowden cable" that operated the choke on old-time cars (See Bowden Wires).

This flexible push-pull cable is available from the manufacturer in many lengths. (It cannot be altered to size by the customer.)

Maintenance The nature of cable usage keeps it exposed to sun and weather, and frequent visual inspection is advised. Check for degrading at the connections of the cable to its load. Look for misalignment and bending. Check for corrosion, for separation of the jacket from its swaged end ferrules. Is the jacket being damaged by rubbing against something? Have jacket bubbles formed to indicate trouble underneath?

If thorough visual inspection leaves any doubts, both ends of the cable should be unhooked, and the core should be moved back and forth manually. Any interference with smooth, easy motion indicates the need for replacement.

The cable should regularly be cleaned and relubricated according to the manufacturer's instructions.

Crash Pads

Crash pads are simple, home-made gadgets for the emergency stoppage of large leaks or hole-throughs. They are especially suitable for wooden boats, because they may be screwed to the hull. On other boats, the crash pads are jammed into place with broom handles or whatever is available.

A crash pad is a square of plywood covered on one side with sheet foam rubber or similar material. Holes for screws are drilled at the four corners.

Installation Convenient sizes for crash pads are: 6 inches square, 9 inches square, and 12 inches square. An easily worked material is ⅜-inch plywood. The holes at the four corners should just pass the screws to be used. The screw length should extend beyond the foam for ½ inch. (No bedding compound is necessary on the crash pad when it is being installed to stop a leak.)

Cruising Hazards

A whisper of wind, glorious sunshine—perfect weather for boating. That's what it was at cast-off. Now, a few hours later at the 180-degree turnaround point, the weather has closed in, and conditions are getting sticky. Such a changing situation is routine for the experienced skipper who has prepared himself for whatever may come. Here are some guiding cautions:

Following seas: When the sea is moving in the same direction but faster than the boat, pressure is built up against the wide transom that typifies the modern powerboat. When this pressure is directly in line with the

CRUISING HAZARDS

course, it may even yield a slight increase in speed; out of line, the result is a yaw to one side or the other. This requires careful attention by the helmsman, who must counteract the undesired movements. (A double-ender, with its sharp stern, is reasonably immune from the problem.)

Grounding: The best advice on grounding is: "Don't go aground!" A long-handled boathook with a red ring painted at the exact draft of the boat is a good avoidance tool if used assiduously in suspected waters.

At the instant of grounding, place power in neutral; do not instantly apply full reverse. (Reverse will not overcome the instant inertia of the boat, and may kick up ground muck.) Assay the situation. Rocking the boat and applying light reverse may get the vessel off. If the location permits boats to run nearby and make waves, so much the better.

In most cases, such simple measures will separate the hull and the bottom, but when they fail, sterner procedures are in order. These are "kedging" or a strong tow from another vessel; a real, solid grounding may require a combination of both. "Kedging" is an old-time trick. The anchor on its rode is taken as far from the boat as the situation will allow (usually rowed out in a dinghy), and worked into the bottom. Back on the boat, a great heave is now given the rode, while the boat is rocked.

Tide has not been mentioned, but, where it exists, it may alter the whole picture. If the tide is rising, the release of the boat will probably be automatic at the cost of some time. A falling tide may be cheated by very fast release attempts. If these fail, a careful check of boat trim is essential to forestall damage and danger when the water falls below the height needed for noraml flotation.

A light grounding usually will reveal a "pivot point" on which the boat is resting and about which the hull may be swung by poling with an oar or a spar. Such wiggling from side to side is a helpful maneuver.

If matters degenerate to the need for heavy pulling on kedge and/or tow, *beware*. A nylon line under stress is a giant rubber band that can snap back in dangerous fashion. If the flying line terminates in a torn-off deck fitting, the whiplash can be lethal.

A hard grounding may cause a leak in a wooden hull and may require a jury-rig repair to assure safety (see Crash Pads).

Jibing: A jibe may be a simple and safe sailboat maneuver, or an event that can lead to a boom-cracked skull. It all depends whether the jibe is excuted intentionally and under control, or accidentally and out of control.

A jibe takes place when the boat is sailing downwind and the breeze swings the mainsail across to the other side. Properly executed, the jibe is under the control of the helmsman, who gives the order to the crew. The accidental jibe can generally be attributed to inattention by the helmsman who lets the condition sneak up on him.

Fog: Some waters are prone to random fog that closes in without much warning and deprives the skipper of the use of visual aids (see Weather). It is a time when every skipper without radar would gladly trade the farm for one; the desire for a Loran or a direction finder comes a close second.

CRUISING HAZARDS

The fogbound skipper has an urgent requirement and two choices. The requirement is for an exact plot of his position on the chart. The choices are either to anchor or to proceed dead slow. The fog signal is kept sounding regardless, and a lookout/"hearout" is stationed at the bow. The need for noise to advertise the presence of the fogbound boat is paramount, whether the noisemaker be a horn giving Coast Guard–approved signals or a heavy spoon banging on a frying pan. In most cases, unless the boat is in open deep water, the better part of valor is to get out of the freeway and tie securely to the ground.

The human mind reacts strangely when fog closes in, and landmarks may be "seen" that are simply not there. A skipper must train himself to resist these imaginings, and he must kill the temptation to steer by them. A distrust of the compass often follows, and this can be fatal. Only experience can eliminate the stomach butterflies that arrive with the woolly fog.

Head seas: Often, the sea and the course many be running in directly opposite directions and the boat is taking a pounding. While a good boat can take more punishment than the people in it, good seamanship and common sense urge an easing of the situation.

The worst pounding will occur when the boat is cutting straight into the sea at speed. Therefore, easing the angle of attack or lowering the speed, or both, will make the ride more comfortable. Timing also helps by synchronizing forward speed with the approach of the waves. (Most of these adjustments are second nature to a skipper thoroughly acclimated to his ship.)

Inlets: Imagine a short section of large-bore pipe at the bottom of a tank to fill and drain it. This is the facsimile of an inlet. Water may be flowing in either direction, or it may be at rest. The only inlet characteristics missing in this illustration are varying depths of water and a partially obstructing sandbar.

It is clear from the example that a boat running an inlet may be going with or against the tide or even traveling unhindered at the stand of the tide. Which of these conditions exists determines the relative difficulty of the passage. The sandbar confuses the wave formation, and generates the major hazard. The presence or absence of breakers at the the sandbar may become the main factor in the decision to run the inlet or heave-to outside and wait.

Here, again, timing becomes an important tool in seeking comfort and safety. The wave formation should be observed to determine the number of waves in a train and their regularity. Boat speed is then adjusted to synchronize as closely as possible. Whether the tide is ebbing or flooding also affects comfort level, with the choice going to the latter.

The big advantage of being on the inside of the inlet is that the trip may easily be canceled if things look ominous. If there are commerical fishermen using the inlet, their attitude toward making the run should form a good guide.

Trim: The forward and aft distribution of weight will determine how the boat behaves when bucking a heavy sea. Rearranging the weight is done by moving passengers and supplies to their most effective positions.

Too much weight too far forward

DAVITS

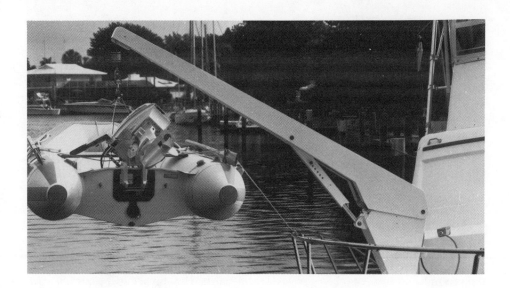

DAVITS—This handsome davit encloses an electric winch. The low-profile design is constructed of aluminum plates. *(Courtesy Mar-Quipt)*

can cause the bow to dive—even to dive severely enough to take in water over the bow. Too much weight too close to the stern can cause a squatting condition that makes for slow response. (See Trim Tabs.) Passengers should stay put. (They usually do, because they are scared.)

PFDs: The wise skipper breaks out the personal flotation devices before the weather gets heavy. True, a PFD can be uncomfortable, but it is effective life insurance. The smartest procedure is to wear a PFD on board at all times (See Personal Flotation Devices.)

Davits

A davit is a vertical metal pipe fastened to the deck or the bulwark at its lower end and with its upper end curved forward to accept a block (See Blocks). A "strongback" (reinforcement) usually is welded across the curve to strengthen it. Davits are commonly found on medium-sized and larger boats. When used for handling the anchor, davits are at the bow; when used for shipping the dinghy, they are located elsewhere, usually at the stern.

Installation The pipe is generally between 1½ and 2½ inches in diameter heavily galvanized. Preferably, the fastening method permits the davit to turn to the best line-up with its load. Where turning is not required, the bottom of the davit may be threaded to a floor flange for solid fastening to the deck. The curved end also often is threaded to a pipe cap that can accommodate a bolt or hook for hanging the blocks.

The dinghy davits should be located at a point where the weight of the load does not seriously heel the boat.

The davit described above is, of course, the home-made version that may be ordered at any plumbing shop. The commercially produced davit is fancier and universally adaptable to ship's chores; it is also several times more expensive. The staid, plain-Jane deck profile created by the bent-pipe davits may be replaced quickly and easily by a moderate investment in today's davit designs. These handsome dinghy-lifters are built around aluminum or stainless box frames immensely stronger than pipes. Operation may be manual, electrical, or hydraulic.

When not in use, the modern davit crouches low on the deck and does not spoil the boat's graceful lines. When there is work to be done, these davits rise to operational height and extend themselves to the required reach. Lifting capacity extends into the range of light outboards.

With extended reach lifting, these davits transmit tremendous torsional stress to the deck area to which they are fastened. This requires extensive through-bolting with backing plates.

The stresses and strains involved between davit and deck may be visualised as a greatly magnified version of what happens when a claw hammer pulls out a headed nail. Remember that the further out the beam of the davit, the greater the stresses occurring for a given load.

Maintenance A davit may be overloaded unintentionally, especially when a power winch becomes part of the hauling system, and care should be taken to avoid this. The overload is more likely with the anchor than with the dinghy.

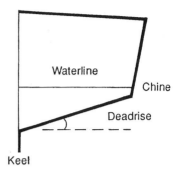

Deadrise

The angle, in section view, between the hull bottom and the waterline (or chine of a V-bottomed boat) is called the "deadrise." It is expressed in degrees and refers to the general line of the bottom (the deadrise angle may bary in degree from bow to stern). For reference, consider a flatbottomed boat: it has zero deadrise. A high-speed, V-bottomed planing hull may have a deadrise exceeding even 20 degrees.

A so-called deadrise boat is stable and comfortable because the rise of the bilge allows the hull to cut through the waves.

Depthsounders

Depthsounders, perhaps more familiarly known by most skippers as "fish finders," use concentrated bursts of high-frequency sound to achieve their results. The bursts are directed to the bottom, and the return echo from any

DEPTHSOUNDERS

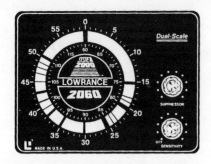

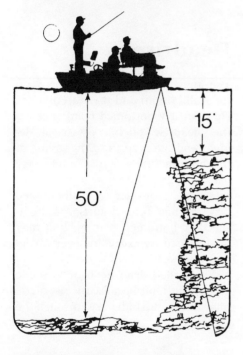

DEPTHSOUNDERS—Shown is a pictorial explanation of the conditions indicated by the depthsounder reading. *(Courtesy Lowrance Electronics)*

intervening target brings back the desired information. The display of the information may be on a screen, on a paper graph, or as a blip on a calibrated scale. The sought-for target between boat and water bottom is a fish.

The function of a depthsounder is best explained by dividing its activity into five areas: (A) generating the high-frequency electrical wave; (B) turning the wave into sound and broadcasting it; (C) receiving the echo and changing it back to an electrical wave; (D) amplifying this echo wave; and (E) displaying the equivalent result as fishing information. The water bottom thus may be shown as a blip on the simpler fish finders and as a topographic line on the more complicated ones, with fish blips above.

The (A) section of the depthsounder is a solid-state oscillator fixedly tuned to a chosen frequency in the range of 50 to 200 kilohertz. A sound at this pitch is beyond the hearing ability of humans. One factor in the choice of the frequency is the maximum depth at which the depthsounder is to be used; the lower frequencies are for the deeper readings. The power developed in these frequencies is expressed as "peak-to-peak watts," actually about eight times the actual RMS (root mean square) watts. As with any transmission, the more power, the greater the penetration of the water. Note that (B) and (C) are one and the same both sound.

The transducer (B) receives the electrical wave from (A) and turns it into sound, much as a loudspeaker would. The design of the transducer causes the sound waves to maintain the shape of a cone with its base on the water bottom. Any fish within that cone, and the bottom as well, will send echoes back up.

The same transducer is (C) as well, functioning in the double capacity of transmitter and receiver. The transducer changes electrical energy into sound and sound energy into electrical

DEPTHSOUNDERS

energy; see Transducer.) Now the various sound echoes are transformed back into electrical waves and are sent on to (D), an amplifier. The strengthened electrical signal now needs only some form of display to make its information available to the skipper. The display (E) is largely determined by the cost and quality of the depthsounder.

The simplest, most popular, and least expensive display is a neon blip on a calibrated circular scale. In the absence of fish, one blip will appear at a point on the scale equivalent to the depth of the water. Fish will generate additional blips above this. A more advanced display will be seen on a liquid crystal screen. Now the actual bottom contour is shown, with any projecting trees or shrubs, plus all fish within the cone. The same picture would appear on a recording depthsounder, except that now there is a permanent record on paper.

Manufacturers have made many improvements in the visibility of the "message" in sunlight and at night. Operating the instrument ranges from turning it on with its switch to selecting from a series of buttons for various specialized results. One model apes a computer by presenting step-by-step instructions on what the operator must do for a desired reading. Some models have pressurized nitrogen within their cases to prevent fogging.

The screen for displaying the information being received by the echoes is a liquid crystal matrix of individual dots called "pixels." The greater the number of pixels, the better the resolution or clarity of the "picture." (It should be emphasized that this is not TV and that groups of blips substitute for actual pictures.)

Most screen-and graph-type fish finders draw a line to separate the bottom from fish resting there. This separation technique is important to fishermen because without it, even large fish would blend into the bottom unseen. A common trade name for this feature is "white line."

Transducers are available in wide variety for in-hull mount, through-hull mount, and transom mount. They may also be selected on the basis of the frequency (in kilohertz) to which they are resonant. The frequency of tranducer and transmitter must be exactly identical for most effective power transfer and maximum depth ability. Some suppliers provide an extra service by tuning the two units to each other before shipment.

The characteristics of the transducer fix the angle of the cone of sound they produce. The sharper the cone, the more thorough the search of the water; a wide cone "views" a greater bottom area.

There is some opportunity to exercise personal choice in the manner in which the depthsounder announces its depth finding. Simplest is the strip of light on the rotating dial. At the other end of the offered instruments is the voice of announcement. (This gives the lone fisherman some "company.") Very popular is the digital indication of water depth. As already mentioned, the printed paper tape provides a permanent record. The numerical accuracy of all models depends on quality of manufacture which, in turn, is governed by price.

Installation Careful and technically correct installation of the transducer is an important prelude to satisfactory operation of the depthsounder. Skip-

DIESEL FUEL

pers loath to drill a hole in the boat bottom have the option of installing the transducer inside. It is not a recommened option. This installation is complicated by the need for a water box, and the sensitivity of the sounder is reduced an amount that depends on the type of hull. The water box is literally a box containing water, fastened tightly to the inside of the hull. The tranducer is placed inside this box. The passage of sound from the box water through the hull and into the outside water is made with minimal loss.

The normal and popular installation of the transducer is through the hull. The required hole is less than 1 inch in diameter and should be located as far astern as needed to get the quietest water and constant immersion at all speeds. The spacing from the keel should be just enough to allow the cone of sound to get by without being cut. The transducer neck should be absolutely vertical, and a fairing block may be needed to achieve this. Liberal use of compounds and proper tightening of nuts should ensure against leakage. The cable run from transducer to depthsounder should be protected. (See also Transducers.)

Maintenance Maintenance consists of keeping the transducer free of fouling. Most manufacturers recommend a light coating of antifouling paint. The trick is to achieve intimate contact of transducer face and water without an air film.

Depth measurement is essentially a measurement of time, the time it takes a sound wave to reach a certain depth and return, and the "clock" for doing this is part of the circuitry and beyond the user's control.

Troubleshooting There is not much in the way of troubleshooting that a skipper can do with a depthsounder when it fails. The options seem to be only checking the continuity of the wiring and cable, cleaning off corrosion, and proving the presence of the necessary voltage with a trouble lamp. Running aground and damaging the transducer are causes to consider.

Repair No part of a depthsounder is self-repairable.

Diesel Fuel

It is startling and difficult to believe, but it is true: Various animalcules, bacteria, microbes, and fungi live happily in diesel fuel. Their "happiness" does not carry over to the skipper, because these living contaminants can block fuel systems and stop engines. Luckily, bactericides are available that kill the offenders and prevent regrowth.

The bactericide is added to the diesel fuel tank in the quantity specified by the manufacturer's instructions. A heavily infested tank may have collected so much bacterial waste matter that the chemical treatment alone is not enough; thorough clean-out now is necessary. The waste most likely is corrosive and harmful to the tank. (Some marinas have treated diesel fuel.)

Gasoline has its octane number, and diesel fuel has its cetane number. The higher the cetane number, the more ignitable the diesel fuel; hence, cetane is a number to check when at the fuel dock. A cetane of 50 is a good grade. (Pure cetane is rated 100).

Diesel fuel is produced by the distillers in three grades: No. 1, No. 2, and No. 3. The numbers are indicative of the "pour point," with No. 1 pouring at the lowest temperature. At temperatures below the pour point, the fuel gets cloudy, the self-contained wax begins to crystallize, and the ability to pour stops. (Obviously this is of little interest to boatmen who inherently are warm-weather diesel fuel buyers.)

At 140,000 Btus per gallon, diesel fuel contains approximately 10 percent more energy than gasoline. Add to this the fact that a diesel engine uses fuel more efficiently than a gas engine, and diesel economy becomes increasingly evident. The added safety of diesel is a tremendous bonus.

A factor in economy is the wide range of fuel/air mixtures that the diesel engine can burn. The amount of fuel shot into the cylinder is directly proportional to the load, and becomes a very high ratio of air to fuel during light duty. By contrast, the gasoline engine is best at its steady diet of 14.7 ration, regardless of load. (In today's market, price per gallon of diesel versus gasoline no longer is an economy source.)

Water is the most likely contaminant in fuel to cause trouble during normal boating. This is not an indictment of the fuel supplier. Almost without exception, the water is the result of condensation in the fuel system. Warm, damp air strikes a cool surface, and the water vapor turns to water. Even a few drops can be disastrous. A water separator that removes the water before the fuel reaches the engine is a sure solution to the problem. (A filter and a water separator may be combined; see Filters.)

Diesel fuel should be chosen on the basis of the lowest percentage of sulfur it contains; some sulfur is inherent. Sulfur combines to form corrosive substances injurious to tanks, piping systems, and engines. Sulfur content should stay below ½ percent.

Maintenance Fuel tank maintenance should include continuous closure of the filler cap to prevent entrance of moist air and foreign matter, and careful check and clean-out of filters and water separators.

Keeping the tank topped up is the best insurance against moisture.

Diodes

Diodes are the simplest of the semiconductor devices (see Transistors). Diodes consist of chips of two rare minerals, held in face-to-face contact and enclosed in a protective housing often half the size of a pea. Power diodes, such as those found in alternators and battery chargers, are, of course, larger and huskier to enable them to handle the high amperage (See Alternators, Chargers).

A diode may be likened to a one-way check valve in a water line. The diode permits electrical currents to flow in only one direction. This is equivalent to converting alternating current to direct current—hence the diodes in alternators and chargers. (Note: The changing of alternating current to direct current is called "rectification.")

Direction Finders (RDFS)

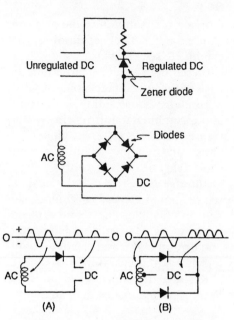

DIODES—The diode is a one-way electrical "gate". How diodes are connected in order to act as "rectifiers" for changing AC to DC in battery chargers and similar devices is shown in these diagrams. (A) and (B) show the half-wave and full-wave modes and the resulting wave forms. The "bridge" connection is the most efficient. The "Zener" diode is a voltage-sensitive regulator.

The "isolators" in multi-battery banks are merely diodes whose one-way characteristic keeps a charged battery from sending its current back to a discharged one. Numbers of tiny diodes are to be found in almost every electronic circuit. The diode is a two-terminal component.

Maintenance Diodes are rated by the peak inverse voltage they can withstand without breaking down. This voltage must never be exceeded. For very high voltages strings of diodes may be connected in series.

The direction finder was the first navigational instrument based on radio science to become available to the skipper. It allowed him to home in on a distant radio transmitter regardless of weather conditions. Best of all, the radio direction finder required no technical knowledge and it was easy to operate.

The market offers radio direction finders (RDFs) in two types: manual and automatic. The difference lies in the manner of seeking the guiding transmitter. The operator of the manual unit must turn the search knob slowly while watching an indicator for the null that indicates a suitable lock-on and presents a reading in degrees. The automatic instrument does this without operator aid. In both cases, the target radio transmitter is first selected, perhaps from a chart.

What makes the scheme work is the directional characteristics of certain radio receiving antennas (see Antennas). This facility is amplified in direction finder antennas by technical design. Often, as in transistor radios, the directivity is there, although not wanted. (In an emergency, a transistor radio can become a crude direction finder by pointing it and noting the change in reception.)

The antennas used in early radio direction finders were large, rotatable loops, commonly seen at the time on the wheelhouses of commercial vessels. The antenna found internally in today's standard direction finder is called a "loop stick." It consists of a powdered iron core on which is wound

DIRECTION FINDERS (RDFS)

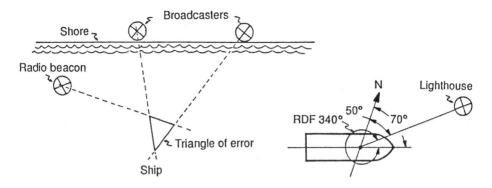

DIRECTION FINDERS (RDFs)—The radio finder easily provides a good fix. The azimuth angle to the target may be measured in reference to several set points. Based on true north, the angle is "true." Based on the compass, the angle is "compass." Based on ship's heading, the angle is "relative." Any system may be used, provided it is maintained throughout.

To get a fix, the azimuth of a target is measured and laid down on the chart as a "line of position." Ditto for a second target. Where the LOPs cross is the fix. A third target results in a fix of greater accuracy because it provides a "triangle of error" within which the ship is located.

a fine-wire inductance. It is sensitive and highly directive. It is the part that turns when the direction finder is searching. (One of today's more advanced direction finders uses an external antenna composed of four small whips set vertically at the corners of a square; see Adcock Antenna.)

The loop stick has one innate failing: It cannot differentiate between reciprocal bearings. The null that indicates "directly ahead" could just as easily mean "directly astern." Luckily, the sense antenna eliminates the ambiguity. The sense antenna is a short whip that is switched into the circuit when there is doubt; by an adding/subtracting routine, it identifies the true reading.

Just as the magnetic compass is deviated by onboard iron, so the radio direction finder may be thrown off by metallic rigging and other metallic masses that reflect, absorb, and reradiate radio waves. Once the best location for the direction finder is chosen, it is worthwhile to make an RDF deviation table like the one for the compass but ignoring magnetism; see Compasses. (It may be possible to find a spot on the boat where a hand-held radio direction finder is free of deviation.)

As is true of most of Nature's functions, the travel of radio waves is not as perfect as it might be, and this affects the accuracy of radio direction finder bearings. These errors arise externally to the boat and are not correctible aboard. Bearings taken at night are "looser" by several degrees than the same would be if taken by day. Another "looseness" occurs when the radio wave being received has traveled close to and parallel to a shore. This ambiguity may reach several degrees.

The standard, lower-cost radio direction finder tunes to the broadcast band and to the transmissions from aids to navigation. The more modern, more accurate RDF receives the VHF band (see VHF-FM Radio). This allows it to function under better all-weather conditions and to tune in NOAA weather transmitters. These may also have a digital readout of direction to target instead merely showing the null.

Installation Several methods of use present themselves to the skipper with an RDF. The unit may become an actual steering aid; it may be used for position finding; and, of course, it is a good-quality radio receiver. The job of installation should include the making of a deviation table with input every 10 or 15 degrees. The preferred situation for doing this has a radio station within sight.

A popular application of the RDF is "homing in." The RDF dial is locked at zero to bring the null forward and parallel with the boat's lubber line (see Compasses). The boat now is swung until a null forward is reached. The helmsman continues to steer to maintain the null. (Extremely cautious watch is kept because the target, or a hazard, may be closer than expected.)

The radio direction finder may also supply lines of position (LOPs). The RDF indicator is assumed to have been installed with zero to the bow. The null is found, and the deviation correction is made. The true ship's bearing is added. The resultant degree inclination is laid down on the chart. Where two (preferably three) LOPs cross is the ship's position, a "fix."

Fluency in using the radio direction finder is gained by practice. As with radar, this practice is most helpful in fine weather when the targets may be observed visually as well as electronically.

Maintenance If the RDF has its own internal battery and is not connected to the 12-volt system, then intermittent checking of the flashlight cells is the only maintenance required. The current drawn by transistor circuits is so low that the cells approach their shelf life; this is especially true of the alkaline cell.

Displacement/ Planing

All powerboat hulls fall into either of two classes: They are displacement hulls or planing hulls—although some modern designs may borrow from both styles. As a general rule, the speedboats are planing hulls. Yet it should be noted that all hulls become displacement hulls when at rest. (Sailboats are displacement hulls.)

Displacement hulls travel *in* the water, while planing hulls try to run *on* the water. The difference is achieved by making use of the hydrodynamic lift generated by the combination of hull design and speed. The reactions between the passing water and the planing hull is like the reaction between the air and the wing of an airplane.

A hull moving through the water in displacement mode creates a bow wave and a quarter wave. The distance between the two increases with speed until its length is equal to the waterline length of the hull. That speed is the theoretical top speed of that displacement hull and, mathematically, is 1.3 times the square root of the waterline. (The length is in feet and the speed is in knots.) The bow wave now becomes a "hump" blocking the bow of the displacement hull from further speed increase.

By contrast, when the planing hull reaches this speed, it has already developed sufficient lift to "go over the hump" and get whatever terminal speed its design and its engines permit. Less and less of its hull is immersed as its speed imcreases. (The truly fast planers appear to be riding on air.)

The lift-generating features of planing design are the shape of the hull and carefully placed, specially shaped lift strakes. The underlying theory mirrors that of aircraft. The changing angle of attack between hull and water as displacement becomes planing often introduces propeller problems.

Doppler Effect

The story may be apocryphal, but it is, nevertheless, an excellent explanation of the "Doppler effect." It seems that Herr Doppler was waiting at a railroad crossing for a train to pass. The train whistle was sounding from before the crossing continuously until some time after.

The ever-alert Doppler noticed that the pitch of the whistle was higher as the train approached, became normal for the few seconds the train remained at the crossing, and then dropped to a lower pitch as the train sped on. This higher-normal-lower pitch sequence is the crux of the Doppler effect. This phenomenon takes place with all wave motion, be it sound, radio, or light. The Doppler effect is the operating basis for many scientific instruments and speed-measuring devices, and the center null is used in satellite navigation to detect the closest approach to the vessel of the orbiting body (see Satellite Navigation Systems). In this usage, the null is the midpoint in the frequency of a radio transmission from the satellite. A Doppler radar gun is used in measuring boat speed during sea trials.

The Doppler effect is easy to understand from a purely logical basis. With the train rushing toward him, Doppler received more sound waves per second, in effect a higher pitch. With the train speeding away, fewer sound waves reached him per second, a lower pitch. With the train at the crossing, the number of waves was simply the normal pitch.

The radar speed gun, much used in checking out the performance of boats, is a Doppler device. It is aimed at the approaching vessel, and speed is read from a dial.

Dynamometers

A dynamometer is a machine for absorbing the power output of an engine and measuring its ability to do work. The energy expended by the engine into the dynamometer is usually dissipated as heat into air or water.

ELECTRICITY

Dynamometers take many forms, from simple to complex. In the simplest form, the test engine drives a generator whose output circuit consists of heavy-duty heating elements. A voltmeter and an ammeter are in the wiring to monitor power levels. Some type of speed indicator keeps tab on rpm.

Output tabulations list the revolutions per minute and the consequent volts and amperes. The nonelectrical factors such as oil pressures and temperature may also be listed during the test.

The volts multiplied by the amperes gives watts, and 746 watts are equivalent to 1 horsepower. Note that this result is a purely theoretical figure that has not taken account of losses.

Dynamometers may also be entirely mechanical. One such is the "pony brake," a true workhorse of the past. In this, the test engine drives a wheel against whose rim a weighted friction shoe is acting as a brake. The weight required to hold a given speed, multiplied by the radius of the wheel, multiplied by the rpm, is the equivalent foot-pounds per minute (33,000 foot-pounds equal 1 horsepower).

$$I = \frac{E}{R} \qquad E = I \times R \qquad R = \frac{E}{I}$$

$R = X + Y$

$L = X + Y$

$C = \frac{1}{X} + \frac{1}{Y}$

$R = \frac{1}{X} + \frac{1}{Y}$

$L = \frac{1}{X} + \frac{1}{Y}$

$C = X + Y$

ELECTRICITY—These three arithmetical statements of Ohm's Law allow electrical problems to be quantified easily. Example: A 2-ohm load is placed on the 12-volt battery circuit. How much current will it draw? ("I" is current in amperes, "E" is voltage in volts, "R" is resistance in ohms.) Answer: $I = \frac{E}{R}, I = \frac{12}{2}, I = 6$ amps. Similarly, "E" and "R" could be solved if unknown. The effects of placing resistance, capacitances, and inductances in series and parallel are explained by these diagrams.

Electricity

Except for the smallest daysailers, electricity in some form is aboard every boat, and thus it behooves the skipper to become familiar with it. Electricity is a willing slave, but it can turn into a dangerous demon when it is mishandled. Yet the rules of correct procedure are simple and sensible.

Electricity is classified by its voltage and to some extent also by the available amperage. The voltage of a circuit is analagous to the pressure in a water line, while the amperage could be considered similar to the amount of water discharged. A flashlight single cell has a voltage of 1½, an automobile storage battery has a voltage of 12, a home lighting circuit is at 120 volts, and the kitchen stove voltage is 220. The current available from the flashlight cell is

ELECTRICITY

a fraction of an ampere, while the storage battery may provide hundreds of amperes.

There are two kinds of electric current: direct current (DC) and alternating current (AC). With direct current, one wire is always positive, the other always negative; batteries deliver direct current. With alternating current, each wire changes its polarity back and forth from positive to negative at a frequency of 60 times per second, or 60 hertz.

(When faced with a circuit of an unknown kind, a simple trick may be used to determine whether it is DC or AC: Dip the two bared wires of the circuit into a glass of salted water. Hydrogen gas will evolve only at the negative pole of a DC circuit but at both wires of an AC circuit.)

Electrical devices may be connected together in either of two ways: either in "series" or "parallel." The series connection takes positive to negative to positive, etc., like a line of elephants that marches tail to trunk. The parallel connection ties all the positives together and all the negatives together.

Simple rules govern the two forms of interconnection. The series system adds the voltages of all the units but keeps the current as of a single unit. The parallel system keeps the voltage as of a single unit and adds the amperages of the units. As an example: The automobile storage battery is composed of six cells in series, each of 2 volts, and the total battery voltage is 12; the available amperage is that of one cell.

The 12 volts from the battery is shockless, but it could release sufficient amperage in a short circuit to heat the wiring red hot and start a fire. In contrast, the 120-volt AC circuit is dangerous, especially in the marine environment, and requires great care; the 220-volt AC is even more so. Remember that salt water is a good conductor of electricity. (See Wiring Code.)

The great advantage of alternating current is that it will function in a transformer (see Transformers). This means that one voltage may easily be transformed into another. Chances are that the marina gets its electric current at a high voltage and transforms it down to the 120 and 240 of the pier outlets. Note that one leg of these 120/240 circuits is always "grounded," that is, connected to the earth and the water. Coming in contact with the "hot" pier wire while standing in a moist location could be fatal.

The passage of electric current through a wire creates a surrounding magnetic field. The existence of this field makes possible electric motors, transformers, loudspeakers, and myriads of other electromagnetic devices. This field is also the reason why the compass is affected by nearby current-carrying electric wires. (Luckily, this undesired effect may be neutralized by twisting the two wires together.) The field from a wire carrying DC current is steady; that from AC current vibrates and interchanges its direction continuously. Transformers need this continuous interchange to function; hence, they may be used only with alternating current. A transformer consists of two independent coils of wire, one the primary, the other the secondary, on a common iron core.

Like magnetic poles repulse each other; unlike poles attract. An electric motor turns because of the repulsive and attractive forces between the sta-

ELECTRICITY

tor and the rotor. The DC motor arranges these necessary forces with its brushes and commutator. The AC motor can function without both commutator and brushes and is therefore simpler in construction.

The voltage of choice (and practicality) on a small boat is 12 volts, because the wide automotive use of this voltage makes equipment reasonable in cost and widely available. The immediate source of power is the storage battery that, in turn, is charged by an engine-mounted alternator or generator. Without an onboard engine, charging is by converted shore power while tied to a pier. (See Alternators and Chargers.)

Large boats retain the 12-volt system for engine starting and add generator or alternator sets driven by their own diesel or gas engines. The low-voltage battery system may include running lights and emergency lighting. The separate generating equipment adds 120-volt and 240-volt alternating current to the ship system for services like those at home. (Note that the common household voltage generally called "110" or "120" is usually 117 volt.) The independent generating sets are rated in kilowatts, "kilo" meaning 1,000.

There is a tendency to regard electric current from an engine-mounted alternator as something "free"—and, of course, Nature gives nothing for free. Such an alternator easily can absorb 1 horsepower from engine output when under full load. And that means an equivalent in extra fuel.

Gasoline- or diesel-powered generators and alternators are not the only means of providing ample electric current aboard pleasure boats. Wind chargers and solar panels have been tried. One difficulty is that the propeller for a wind charger must be large if worthwhile electric current is to be obtained. Obviously, such a prop has no place on a small boat. Likewise, presently available solar panels occupy much space and deliver less than 1 ampere in sunlight; at best, this could be only a "trickle" charge for the battery.

Some accessory equipment is rated in "watts." One watt is the product of one ampere multiplied by one volt. This relationship is true in DC circuits. It is not strictly true in AC circuits but yet is close enough for valid approximations.

Installation An electrical installation with several branches should originate in a switch panel. Any synthetic sheet, approximately ⅜ inch thick and cut to the required rectangular size, makes a good panel. This panel should be mounted sturdily in a naturally dry location with access to front and back. Switches, meters, circuit breakers, fuses are all mounted on the panel front in closely related groups.

The question arises: Fuses or circuit breakers? Both devices must be bought for a finite amperage, and their protection extends only over a narrow range. The circuit breaker is reset after every break; the fuse is thrown away after a "break". The cost of a circuit breaker is many times that of a fuse. Cost and convenience therefore are the bases for a decision. (See Circuit Breakers, Fuses.)

Maintenance Maintenance in electrical circuits consists of keeping all connections tight and free of corrosion.

ELECTROLYSIS

Troubleshooting The voltohmmeter and the trouble lamp are the troubleshooting tools (see Voltohmmeter and Trouble Lamps).

Repair Repairing electrical circuits requires a soldering iron and insulating tape (see Soldering). An insulation stripper becomes really handy.

Electrolysis

Whenever two different metals are placed in an electrolyte (and salt water is an excellent electrolyte), an electric cell is formed. If the two metals are connected with an electric wire, current will flow, and one of the metals will waste away. How fast this will take place depends on how close to each other the two metals are placed on the galvanic scale. This scale puts magnesium at one end and platinum at the other. The metal nearer magnesium will be the positive anode, and the metal nearer platinum becomes the negative cathode.

Magnesium is more active than desired, and the next metal, zinc, is considered to be the end of the galvanic scale for boatyard and practical purposes. Zinc, in appropriate form, is attached to underwater metal for the purpose of sacrificing itself and thereby protecting the metal against "electrolysis," the name for the wasting process. The zinc must be chemically pure in order to be effective; commercial zinc will not do the job. (See also Zincs.)

Theory and practice on electrolysis protection do not always agree. As a result, zince often is found where it is not necessary or else in greater amount than needed. Boatyards have found that zinc is a good source of profit on material and on the labor to install it.

Theoretically, a boat with shaft, propeller, rudder, and struts of the same metal does not need zinc. An exception arises when the metal is an alloy whose ingredients are far enough apart galvanically to cause electrolytic self-destruction. In such a case, zinc overrides the chemically generated current and protects.

The immersed metals to be protected must be tied together electrically and to the zinc. An unconnected underwater metal will receive no protection. The connection may consist of copper wire or copper strip. The zinc must remain unpainted and unfouled.

To show how theory may often leave areas of doubt, consider two boats tied to a pier. Each boat has all systems grounded as per the best instructions, and each has taken shorepower cable aboard. One boat has an aluminum propeller, while the prop on the other boat is bronze. An analysis of the situation reveals that the two propellers are now connected together with low-resistance, excellent-conductivity shore cable. An electrolytic cell has been formed with bronze, aluminum, and salt water, and an electric current is being generated. Given time, the aluminum propeller will disappear! (It would appear that the theory promulgating universal grounding is not always entirely sound.)

It is possible for an excellent zinc installation to generate enough countercurrent to override the foregoing situation. There is also a method of

ELECTROLYSIS

Galvanic Series of Metals in Sea Water

ANODIC OR LEAST NOBLE—ACTIVE

Magnesium and magnesium alloys
CB75 aluminum anode alloy
Zinc
B605 aluminum anode alloy
Galvanized steel or galvanized wrought iron
Aluminum 7072 (cladding alloy)
Aluminum 5456
Aluminum 5086
Aluminum 5052
Aluminum 3003, 1100, 6061, 356
Cadmium
2117 aluminum rivet alloy
Mild steel
Wrought iron
Cast Iron
Ni-Resist
13% chromium stainless steel, type 410 (active)
50-50 lead tin solder
18-8 stainless steel, type 304 (active)
18-8 3% NO stainless steel, type 316 (active)
Lead
Tin
Muntz metal
Manganese bronze
Naval brass (60% copper—39% zinc)
Nickel (active)
78% Ni.-13.5% Cr.-6% Fe. (Inconel) (Active)
Yellow brass (65% copper—35% zinc)
Admiralty brass
Aluminum bronze
Red brass (85% copper—15% zinc)
Copper
Silicon bronze
 5% Zn.—20% Ni—75% Cu.
90% Cu.—10% Ni.
70% Cu.—30% Ni.
88% Cu.— 2% Zn.—10% Sn. (Composition G-bronze)
88% Cu.— 3% Zn.—6.5% Sn.—1.5% Pb (composition M-bronze)
Nickel (passive)
78% Ni.—13.5% Cr.—6% Fe. (Inconel) (Passive)
70% Ni.—30% Cu.
18-8 stainless steel type 304 (passive)
18-8 3% Mo. stainless steel, type 316 (passive)
Hastelloy C
Titanium
Platinum

CATHODIC OR MOST NOBLE—PASSIVE

ELECTRONIC CONTROL

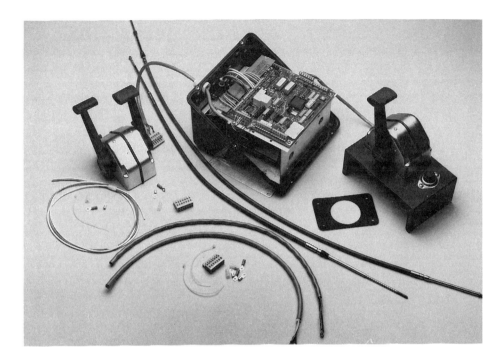

ELECTRONIC CONTROL—Shown are the console levers, the actuator, and the Bowden cables of the Electronic Engine Control. The eight-wire electric cable from console to engine may reach a length of 70 feet. *(Courtesy Mathers Micro Commander)*

avoiding it which requires isolation transformers, one on each boat. Such transformers are heavy, large, and expensive, and therefore little used.

Electrolysis is not restricted to immersed metals but may also take place anywhere differing metals in contact are exposed to spray and rain. A few drops of seepage plus acid and salt from the air can provide sufficient electrolyte. The dissolution of the metal may have gone beyond casual outward appearance and may create a danger due to loss of strength. When dissimilar metals must be together, an insulating washer may help. (When a zinc is attached to a painted surface, the immediately adjoining paint may suffer a "burn" from the passing electric current.)

ELECTROLYSIS—This table predicts the corrosive action on two dissimilar metals connected together and immersed in seawater. The farther apart the metals are in the table, the stronger the action and the greater the degeneration. *(Courtesy American Boat & Yacht Council)*

Electronic Control

Remote control of the engine from the console requires some system of transmitting the exact movement of the console lever. Systems in use employ

EMERGENCY GEAR

oil under pressure, air under pressure, pulleys and cable, Bowden push-pull cables, and others (see Bowden Wires, Controls/Cable). All entail some difficulty in installing the console–cable connection. Now an "electronic engine control" (more accurately, an electromechanical control) simplifies the installation by running only an electric cable from the console to the engine. (At the engine the action changes from electronic to Bowden cable.)

The heart of this device is the "servo" motor, often called a follower motor because the slave minutely duplicates the rotary position of the master. The terminus of the system at the engine is an "actuator" that moves short Bowden wire cables attached to throttle and reverse gear. Positioning the console throttle is equivalent to positioning the engine throttle. The same console lever also sets the gear for forward, neutral, and reverse. With a twin-screw installation, the engines are automatically synchronized. The design permits up to five remote-control points, with only one "live" at a time. The actuator can exert as much as 40 pounds of effort against the engine and reverse-gear levers.

Installation This control is sensitive to low voltage from the 12-volt boat battery and should not be connected to the starting battery if that may be avoided. Installation and testing are covered fully in the owner's manual.

CAUTION: The electronics of this remote control are susceptible to damage by normal static discharges. Consequently, anyone working on the actuator with the cover removed should wear a static-discharge wrist bracelet.

Emergency Gear

All of the following listed items have been individually helpful in some emergency situation. For his own future protection each skipper should choose those items that fit the boat and his style of cruising:

• Signaling equipment, such as megaphones, bells, horns, flags, pennants, flashlights, and hand-held searchlights.

• Radar reflectors, EPIRBs, strobe lights, flares, manoverboard lights and poles, life rings, buoyancy bags, flotation devices, life rails, and sea anchors.

• Emergency desalinators, rigging cutters, fire extinguishers, personal rescue packs, shark repellants, and sea dye markers.

• Safety apparel, such as safety harnesses, flotation collars, deck shoes, and foulweather gear.

• Sunglasses and sunscreen.

• A large watertight, buoyant bag to carry many of the above items and others, such as a parafoil kite, polypropylene underwear, chemical heaters, and a space (plastic) blanket.

• Gear needed for long-term survival can also include solar stills or water makers, a juicer (to extract moisture from fish), spear gun, fish gaff, fishing line and hooks, cutting board, wire saw, plankton net, and writing materials.

Maintenance Emergency gear should be stored at a location aboard that would be accessible in the worst emergency conditions. Each item should be devoid of wrappings and ready to perform its duty. Devices with batteries should be checked regularly.

ENGINES

(See: EPIRBs, Fire Extinguishers, Life Rails, Personal Flotation Devices, Radar Reflectors, Sea Anchors, Strobe Lights.)

Engine Overheating

One day the pointer of the temperature indicator may cross the red line that marks the maximum temperature at which the engine is to be run safely. This may or may not be a crisis. The generally low accuracy of small-boat console instruments introduces a measure of doubt: It may be the indicator. The experienced skipper will resort to his in-built "instruments" of sight and touch.

First he uses sight: Is the usual volume of cooling water flowing overboard? Next, touch: Does a finger tip touched to the flow suggest the usual working temperature? If so, no crisis, and the indicator and its sender can be checked or replaced at the pier.

A less happy situation would be clouds of steam around the exhaust flow. The indicator is probably correct in signaling trouble brewing.

Troubleshooting The first check should be for blockage of the cooling-water intake.

The cooling-water pump on an outboard engine usually is not available for spot repairs, but its counterpart on an inboard engine is belt driven. The belt, most likely, is the villain responsible. Carrying an adjustable vee-belt of the correct width permits excellent first aid. The links in these belts may be removed or added to fit the problem at hand. In an emergency, small-sized line may be tied tightly over the two pulleys with sufficient drive resulting to allow slow-speed running, with constant alertness for overheating.

Another possible cause for engine overheating is a locked-up thermostat (see Thermostats). Thermostats are relatively easy of access, and the offender should be removed.

Engine misadjustments alone may be the cause of engine overheating despite correct cooling-water flow. Spark timing that has skipped into major retard is a familiar precursor of overheating. An emergency readjustment may be made without instruments by simply advancing the timing a few degrees. A fairly close setting is possible if the advance is made with the engine running and the position noted that gives highest speed.

Engines

The internal-combustion engine, fueled either by gasoline or by diesel oil, is the common propulsion power plant for pleasure boats. In general, the diesel engine is reserved for the larger vessels.

All internal-combustion engines suck in a mixture of air and fuel, compress it, ignite it, and then turn the resulting release of energy into rotary motion. The output shaft transmits the generated power to the propeller or other means of moving water. The forward motion of the boat is the reaction from the water thrown rearward.

ENGINES

The transition from fuel to released energy is made in either two strokes or four strokes of the piston, depending upon design, and the engine thus becomes a "two-stroke-cycle" or a "four-stroke-cycle" power plant. The two-stroke cycle, with gasoline, is almost entirely reserved for outboard motors, with larger inboard engines using the four-stroke cycle. In the diesel world, large engines are marketed for each mode of operation, and each has its excellent operational record.

A scrutiny of the individual cycles discloses the following: In the two-stroke cycle, the first upward travel of the piston compresses the fuel to make it ready for ignition. The same stroke, by making use of the suction created by the piston bottom (and valves), brings in fuel. Combustion is started at the top of the piston travel, and the resulting high pressure forces the piston down in a power stroke. Again, the bottom of the piston is doing double duty by forcing new fuel into the combustion chamber. Thus, there is a power stroke once in each revolution of the flywheel. (Each stroke is half a revolution.)

In the four-stroke cycle, the power stroke occurs only once in every *two* revolutions of the flywheel. The actions of the piston are greatly simplified.

The first stroke, a downward travel of the piston, creates a suction that draws the fuel mixture into the combustion chamber. Stroke two, upward, compresses the fuel and makes it ready for ignition at the top of the travel. In stroke three, the piston is forced down in its power stroke by the energy released from combustion. The piston's return to the top, stroke four, clears out the burnt gases. The energy retained in the flywheel from the power stroke makes strokes one, two, and four possible. The excess power is delivered to the engine output shaft as rotary motion.

The "traffic cop" for the movements of burnt and unburnt fuel is a system of valves. In the four-stroke-cycle engine they are intake and exhaust valves actuated by a cam shaft and minutely timed to piston travel. The two-stroke-cycle engines generally use flapper valves that respond to the pressures and suctions of piston travel. Often, ports in the cylinder wall that are covered and uncovered by the piston are used.

The comparatively small cross section of a valve opening becomes an impediment to the fast gas movement required by a high-speed engine. To overcome this, designers may double or triple the number of valves per cylinder.

Because it takes a specific amount of time for the flame to travel, ignition must take place prior to the arrival of the piston at top dead center. This lead time is known as "advance timing." It is one of the variables that is adjusted during "tune-up." A ballpark figure of the timing used for an average propulsion engine is 20-odd degrees before top dead center; the owner's manual is the final word (see Ignition).

The ratio of fuel to air in the mixture fed to the gasoline engine is critical and is maintained by a correctly adjusted carburetor. Only minimal departures from the optimum ratio are "accepted" by the gas engine. Such departures include "choking," an extra-

ENGINES

rich mixture for starting a cold engine, or a rich shot of fuel for acceleration (see Carburetors).

Outboard motors are built around engines with from one to six cylinders (see Outboard Motors). Inboard engines are designed with four, six, or eight cylinders; the sixes and the eights are generally in the vee form. Many of the larger power plants are so-called "marinized" automotive units; these bring to the boating world the benefits from the many improvements in car and truck power.

Engine horsepower is directed to the propeller through a transmission. This transmission may only provide a clutch and means of reversing the rotation of the output shaft, or it may include gear trains for speed reduction. Unlike automobile transmissions, the marine units are continuously under load, always going "uphill," and must be built accordingly. (See Transmissions). Transmission cooling becomes as important as engine cooling.

A major improvement for all gasoline engines resides in the adoption, by almost all models, of "electronic ignition" (see Ignition). Troublesome breaker points are eliminated, and, best of all, an adjustment in timing does not change with age and wear. This breakerless form of ignition also generates much higher spark-plug voltages with which to combat the moisture-laden marine ambiance.

Maintenance The owner's manual is the best guide to the proper maintenance of a marine engine. As already noted, the marine power plant works under constant load and never gets the opportunity to "coast." Oil therefore assumes an important role (see Lubricating Oils). The number of quarts of oil that constitute a correct filling, and especially the intervals of running hours after which the oil should be replaced, are explained in the owner's manual; likewise, the replacement of filters.

The manual also mandates the working life of spark plugs—but this may be taken with a bit more allowance because of the high quality of modern plugs. The secret lies in the occasional removal of the plugs for common-sense inspection (see Spark Plugs).

This laws of Nature decree that only a small percentage of the energy in the fuel can actually be turned into useful work. The balance goes into waste heat that must be dissipated via a cooling system in order to maintain the engine at a safe temperature. In all but the smallest marine power plants, the cooling medium is continuously circulating water. An important chore of maintenance is keeping the water flow uninterrupted; frequent visual check of the outflow of water should become a habit. (See Thermostats.)

Water cooling of marine engines functions in one of two ways. The water may be drawn in, circulated once through the cooling system, and discharged. This is "raw-water" cooling. Contrarily, the engine may have its coolant permanently locked within it's system, transferring its heat to continuously circulating raw water through a heat exchanger. This is "freshwater" cooling. The advantage of this latter method is the ability to keep anti-rust fluids in the engine.

Checking belt tightness is a maintenance chore. The accepted norm is a

73

ENGINES

maximum deflection of ½ inch when the long expanse is pushed in with the finger (with the engine dead, of course).

The drain hole at the bottom of the oil pan makes it easy to dump oil from an automobile engine. This drain hole loses its usefulness when the engine is installed in a boat, with the pan of necessity in the bilge. Now oil may be drained from the engine only by inserting the pickup tube from a small oil pump into the dipstick opening. Note that oil removal is best done when the oil is still warm from running.

It goes without saying that engine maintenance also includes keeping control levers, wires, pulleys, and whatever, lubricated and free.

Troubleshooting Engine troubleshooting logic: In order to function, an internal-combustion engine requires air, fuel, compression, ignition. The air-and-fuel mix must be in the combustion range. The compression must throw a noticeable load on the starter (a great load, in the case of a diesel). The ignition must be visible with the wires slightly removed from the spark plug (except with a diesel). When one of these necessaries is absent, the problem is obvious; when all are present and yet there is a failure to run, the problem is mechanical.

Like a doctor using a stethoscope, a mechanic may learn much by listening through his own "stethoscope" consisting of a long screwdriver or a short length of heater hose. The blade of the screwdriver is touched to various points of the running engine, and the handle is held to the bone behind the ear. The hose is used similarly. Improper noises from the engine are clearly heard and tell their story.

Key turned, engine does not crank: Low battery. Corroded cables. (See Starters.)

Engine cranks, does not start: No fuel. No ignition. No compression. Timing failure. Flooded engine. (See Carburetors and Ignition.)

Engine runs, but ragged: Fouled spark plugs. Misplaced plug wires. Cross-sparking in distributor cap. Mixture too lean. (See Carburetors.)

No oil pressure indication: Low oil. Excessive bearing clearance. Defective sender or guage. Faulty pump. Oil grade too light. (See Lubricating Oils.)

Engine knocks on load: Fuel octane too low. Timing too advanced. Engine overheated. (See Diesel Fuel, Engine Overheating, Ignition, and Timing.)

Engine suddenly stops: Empty fuel tank. Broken fuel line. Break in ignition circuit. Carburetor fuel filter clogged. Engine without water and seized solid from overheating. Propeller fouled solid. (See Carburetors, Engine Overheating, and Propellers.)

The VOM is the instrument of choice in checking continuity of the electrical circuit and measuring voltage (see Voltohmmeter).

Repair It seems as though designers begrudge the space devoted to power plants and consider it as an area subtracted from passenger enjoyment. As a result, many engines are located in a manner that allows no working space around them. A mechanic attempting a repair onboard can become stymied by poor access. Complete removal of the engine to a shop often becomes necessary. Proper installation should

EPIRBs

permit at least belt changes and tightening, carburetor adjustment, and timing checks.

Overhaul procedures duplicate what is done with automobile engines: valve grinding, cylinder bore work and subsequent ring fitting, bearing insert replacement, usually also spark plug and cable replacement. Compression checks should be made for all cylinders, and the readings should be nearly equal and within the range given in the owner's manual.

Most engine repairs require skill and special tools not available to an average pleasure-bout skipper. Nevertheless, a thorough familiarity with the engine improves the contact with a mechanic.

Carburetors require remarkably little attention besides cleanliness and an unclogged fuel filter (see Carburetors).

EPIRBs

EPIRB is an acronym for Emergency Position Indicating Radio Beacon. In appearance this is a small, tubular canister with a short whip antenna at one end. Its function is to activate itself automatically in an extreme distress situation and then send continuous radio distress signals for rescuers to home in on. Construction is solid state and waterproof.

The three models of EPIRBs available (Class A, Class B, and Class C) have now been joined by a superior Category I whose characteristics add to the chance of successful rescue. Carrying

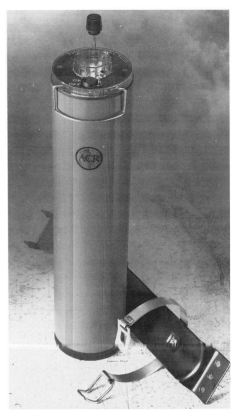

EPIRBs—Shown is a popular EPIRB together with its quick-release holding bracket. Landing in the water activates the device. *(Courtesy ACR)*

an EPIRB is not required by Coast Guard regulations for pleasure vessels, but it is mandated for commercial craft. However, an EPIRB is basic safety equipment for any boat venturing offshore. Purchasers of the Category I unit are required to register their boat with NOAA, together with any details that could facilitate rescue.

Conventional EPIRBs (Class A, Class B, and Class C) transmit on two radio frequencies, 121.5 megahertz and

243.0 megahertz. These frequencies were chosen because they are monitored by aircraft. Experience has found, however, that this monitoring is not reliable enough to be adequate in spotting distress, because of normally heavy radio traffic. Category I EPIRBS transmit on a special frequency of 406 megahertz that is received by satellites of the COMPASS-SARSAT system. The received distress signal is then processed and taken over by the Coast Guard for rescue action.

The output power of the EPIRB radio transmitter is less than 1 watt, but this is sufficient for its mode of operation. The unit must be capable of at least 48 hours' continuous operation, at full output. The Class A and Category I EPIRBS are preferably carried in a holder in an inverted position and in a location where the instrument can float free if the ship sinks. It is then expected to right itself, raise its antenna, and begin transmitting. (Some Class B and Class C EPIRBS are manually launched and activated.)

The advent of the Category I EPIRB, and its special frequency, was made necessary by the inadequacy of the existing system. The Class A EPIRB sent a plain distress signal without identifying characteristics—a signal easily lost in the hubbub of communication traffic. The Category I transmitter has provision for modulation. This modulation consists of the information submitted to the NOAA at the time of purchase. Thus, rescuers immediately know the type of ship they are seeking.

Much of the dissatisfaction with the Class A situation was caused by false alarms. Skippers tested their EPIRBS, or else the devices turned on accidentally. For listeners it became the old story of the cry of "Wolf!" General optimism prevails that the Category I and its 460-megahertz frequency, together with the satellite processing network, will prove a boon to sea rescue.

An overview of the complete EPIRB picture seems to lead to the conclusion that the older units impart a false sense of safety—and that choice should be restricted to the new Category I. This may be a correct conclusion. One difficulty is cost; Category I is much more expensive.

NOTE: The Class B is similar to Class A but is built to less stringent specifications. Class C is another step down. A general summary places Classes A and B in the boats of passagemakers and Class C in coastal vessels—and with Category I supreme for all services.

Maintenance Based on general statistics, the likelihood that the EPIRB will be used in a truly distress situation is small. Consequently, maintenance consists of inspections at reasonable intervals to verify that the device is still fully operable. The manufacturer's instructions should be followed. Batteries generally have a four-year shelf life; the need to replace the batteries may arise.

Repair The construction of an EPIRB eliminates home repair.

Fiberglass

Fiberglass-reinforced plastic (FRP) is the modern wonder material for plea-

FIBERGLASS

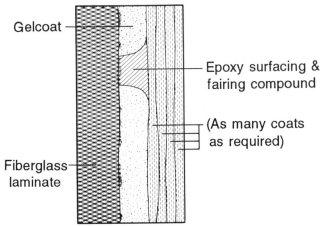

FIBERGLASS—A time comes when the gelcoat of a fiberglass hull is too far "gone" and improvable only with paint designed for that purpose. This cross section shows a fiberglass hull section that has been "faired" (made smooth) and given four coats of paint. Note the filled blister. *(Courtesy Interlux)*

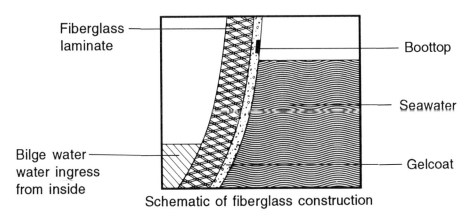

FIBERGLASS—Fiberglass is generally considered waterproof, but in actuality it is permeable by seawater. True, the permeability is microscopic, but over a period of time water sufficient to cause blisters may get through. This cross-section shows the makeup of a representative fiberglass hull. *(Courtesy Interlux)*

sure-boat construction. It has forced time-honored wood almost totally from the field. Wood is Nature's gift to the boatbuilder. It is amenable to any design, and the result depends only on the expertise of the builder. But wood is vulnerable to both rot and infestation, which greatly reduce the allure of the gift. Fiberglass is strong, durable, requires little maintenance, and easily conforms to the beautiful lines of today's designs. Nature has evolved no hungry borers (teredos) to destroy it as they do wood. Fiberglass has made mass-production boats possible at affordable prices.

Although fiberglass occupies center stage in today's boating world, there are many other time-honored and seaworthy methods of boat construction

FIBERGLASS

in use. Among these are wood (both plywood and solid), steel, aluminum, and ferrocement. Modern fiberglass construction is aided by various core materials and may even substitute other resins than polyester, like epoxies.

The fact that fiberglass basically is a highly flexible thread, despite the inclusion of the word "glass," puzzles newcomers. Yet thread it is, spun out from molten glass. This thread is woven and combined into many forms, just as ordinary thread becomes various fabrics. Thus, fiberglass for boat use is available in woven cloth, in mat, in roving, and in tapes. Each of these types of "fabric" fills a special need in boat building and repair.

The name "fiberglass-reinforced plastic" tells the full story of its composition. The plastic (generally based on polyester resin, although epoxy is often used in sheathing a hull or deck) is reinforced with one or more forms of fiberglass materials. The accepted explanation of why this adds strength always cites reinforced concrete: Plain concrete has nominal strength; add internal steel reinforcing rods, and you can build skyscrapers. The resins used in fiberglass boat construction are synthetic marvels of chemistry; the resin gathers its own strength by cross-linking its molecules.

The commercial construction of pleasure boats is either "production" (many duplicates) or "one-off" (only a single boat of that model). The preliminary stages are practically the same for both: An exact model or "plug" is made to the designer's specifications. A mold is made from this plug. The boat hull itself is built up in the mold. The plug's surface must be polished to a perfect high gloss because it, in turn, determines the finish of the mold and subsequently of the hull. If there are re-entrant curves in the design, the mold may need to be made in sections to permit release of the hull.

Construction of the boat hull begins with the application of a release agent to the surface of the mold. The release agent prevents the applied resin from sticking to the mold. The actual hull buildup begins with the subsequent application of the "gelcoat" after the waxy part of the release agent has been polished to a high lustre.

The gelcoat is resin without reinforcement and it usually is pigmented to the color desired for the boat. The wax in the release agent serves the double purpose of preventing the gelcoat from sticking to the mold while permitting the outer face of the gelcoat to attain maximum hardness by shutting it off from the air. The inner exposed face of the gelcoat cures only to a tacky condition that makes an excellent bond to later coats of fiberglass and resin. In "hand layup," these later layers are applied manually.

The strength of the fiberglass hull is a direct result of the number of layers of resin and reinforcement and of the type of material used. Fiberglass is not the only reinforcement commercially in vogue; a core may be included for extra strength, or strong fibers (for instance, graphite) may be added to the mix. The designer orders the required strength by specifying certain materials and a final thickness. Areas of great stress—for instance, a transom to hold an outboard motor—are beefed up, often by adding plywood.

FIBERGLASS

Some old but worthy (although leaky) wooden boats have been saved from the grave with fiberglass. The old hull is treated as a "plug," and the reinforced fiberglass/resin combination is built upon it. To forestall delamination (a possibility with many kinds of wood), the first layers of the coating are stapled to the hull. For all practical purposes, the wooden vessel becomes a fiberglass one with the benefits thereof.

In all fiberglass construction, maintenance, and repair, it is important to respect the chemical limitations of the resins. For instance, never attempt to apply polyester resin over epoxy, because adherence will be unsatisfactory.

Maintenance The maintenance of a fiberglass boat may be summed up as a major operation of cleaning and polishing. In the absence of damage, the gelcoat of a boat and the paint require approximately the same attention with similar cleaning aids. The first step is a thorough wash with fresh water (not with salt water) to which a few squirts of kitchen detergent have been added to act as a wetting agent. This is followed by a thorough waxing with a good boat or automobile wax compound, preferably one that includes an ultraviolet-ray blocker. The final step is buffing the wax to a high lustre, and this may be done manually or with great care with a power buffer.

Slight scratches, abrasions, and discolorations may be rubbed out with auto-body compound that contains an abrasive. The caution here is to remember that an abrasive really removes some surface and to take it easy. When the "end of the line" is reached on what wax and compounds can accomplish, there is always paint, after all wax is removed.

Repair One of the advantages of fiberglass boats is the relative ease with which repairs may be made after minor accidents. Every popular boating area breeds its quota of dents, scratches, and holes, and many of these a handy boatman can repair himself. In most instances, these fixes are purely cosmetic and do not affect the boat's integrity. The materials for making these repairs are readily available in marine stores and at marinas. The illustrations explain how the work is performed.

"Osmotic blistering" is one possible thorn for the owner of a fiberglass boat. Blisters are caused by water seepage through the surface. (Yes, seepage is possible through that apparently impenetrable fiberglass surface.) Several paint companies supply the materials for repair with instructions.

Let common sense be the guide in the matter of gloves, masks, and other protection when working with resins and solvents, and around dust; assure adequate ventilation.

The wax normally in the repair area will prove bothersome unless it is thoroughly removed by washing with acetone. The injured surface then is cut out to a diameter large enough to reach "healthy" fiberglass all around. A long, wide feather edge is sanded evenly around the hole to provide a grip for the application of resin and reinforcement. A temporary closure of the hole (cardboard, aluminum sheet) is fastened in place and becomes the backstop against which the new material is applied. Cellophane sheet is placed so that it will cover whichever

FILTERS (FUEL)

surface will be outside when the work is finished; this reduces curing time and leads to a harder finish more amenable to sanding. A gelcoat mix (resin and pigment) may be used as the final coat where the repair becomes part of the gelcoat of the vessel, but this may turn out to be the more difficult part of the job.

What looks like good fiberglass cloth at a lower price is not necessarily good for fiberglass work. The cloth (mat, roving) that is to be used successfully for boat jobs should be free of wax and should have been treated for maximum resin compatibility. Whether or not a fiberglass is suitable is best determined by its source.

The importance of correct cure times cannot be overstressed. A common amateur mistake is to keep applying the resin after it has started to cure and has lost its initial sticking ability.

Final sanding is an important portion of the repair and, to a large extent, determines final appearance. Wet-and-dry paper, around 300 grit, is recommended, with water as the lubricant. A few strokes with auto-body compound prior to waxing may prove worth the extra toil.

The fiberglass hull has no frames and no floors to tie the frames to the keel; its designed shape is maintained by bulkheads. (The "floors" are not the walk-upon floor of the landlubber, but rather they are connecting pieces between frame and keel.) Usually, these bulkheads are of plywood enclosed in fiberglass.

Note that fiberglassed-plywood shelves may be attached to the bulkheads by "welding" the surfaces with additional resin and 'glass.

The brushes for fiberglass work should be the cheap "throwaway" kind because their active work span will be only the time it takes for the resin/hardener (catalyst) mix to harden. The quality of the job is not affected by the quality of the brush as it is in painting. If the plastic pails for the mix are of the Teflon type, they may be reused because the resin will not stick and may be dumped out after curing.

Filters (Fuel)

Engines, both gasoline and diesel, are vulnerable to tiny bits of foreign matter as well as to water in their fuel. Carburetor jets and injector nozzles become clogged, and the engine limps or stops. Filters are the solution—filters for fuel, filters for oil, filters to take out water, filters for air.

Filters are simple devices. They force the fluid to be filtered through a filtering material whose spaces between fibers are smaller that the contaminant to be removed. (At some point the spaces will be filled and the filter will be blocked and need replacement.) Water separation takes place because of the different surface tensions of water and of fuel, and because of the hydrophobic nature of the filter element. A good filter removes particulate contaminants as small as a micron, one-millionth of one meter. Some filters contain permanent magnets, the better to hold iron and steel particles.

A typical filtering sequence occurs as follows: Large foreign particles are removed; tiny water droplets strike the

FILTERS (FUEL)

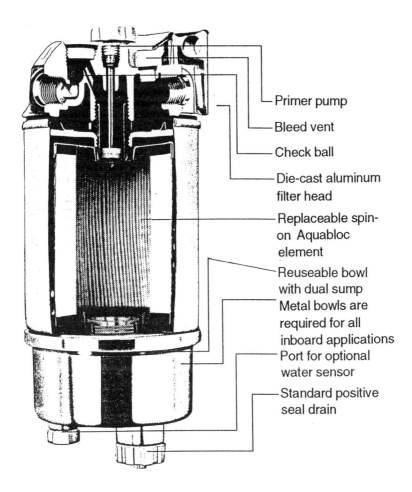

FILTERS—This cut-open view shows what makes a filter filter. *(Courtesy Racor Division)*

filter and coalesce into drops heavy enough to fall into the sump; remaining contaminants are removed down to the rating of the filter; the fluid emerging from the filter is clean and waterless.

A typical commercial filter is the approximate size and shape of a quart oil can. Threaded holes at top and bottom permit the quick "spin-on" of the filter to the engine and of the sump to the filter. The sumps are available in see-through plastic and in metal. (For gasoline engines, the Coast Guard mandates metal.) For in-line installations, a unit with nipples and valves and a primer pump screws onto the top of the filter element can.

Gasoline engines have a nasty habit of backfiring and shooting a flame

FIRE EXTINGUISHERS

from the carburetor air intake. In response, the Coast Guard requires approved flame arresters on the carburetors of all marine gasoline engines. The arrester serves also as an air cleaner and sound deadener. (Caution is advised whenever the engine is run temporarily without the arrester during repairs.)

Installation An excellent installation hooks filters up in pairs. The plumbing and valves allow either filter to be isolated so that the engine may be kept running while a filter examination and substitution are being made. Filter service life is determined by experience with unique local conditions and with suggestions from the owner's manual.

Maintenance The sumps of filters should be checked frequently for water and for debris. When the filter is on a line containing a pressure gauge, the condition of the filter element may be estimated by depreciations in gauge readings.

A clogged flame arrester may enrich the fuel mixture and raise havoc with engine economy and performance.

A water sensor is available for attachment to the sump. This may be wired to the console to send a buzzer or light signal to the skipper when water accrues.

Troubleshooting Water in the fuel is not automatically a demerit for the fuel supplier. Predominantly, the water is there due to the workings of Nature. The damp sea air strikes the cool surface of the tank, and the airborne moisture condenses into water. Keeping the tank topped up to exclude as much air as possible is the only remedy. Adding a "dry gas" fluid may help.

Fire Extinguishers

No emergency that confronts a skipper underway can be as terrifying as fire. The very anomaly of flames at the center of vast quantities of water can add to the likelihood of panic. Survival suddenly depends on the firefighting equipment carried aboard, and on the skipper's ability to use it effectively. If the equipment is automatic, the battle is partially won.

All powerboats and most sailboats carry flammable fluids in the form of fuel for engines and for stoves. Rated in the order of the danger these fluids project, gasoline would head the list; it has often been compared to dynamite. Following in dangerous potential would be tank gases, highly volatile solvents, and diesel oil, the last a comparatively safe giant difficult to ignite. The circumstances create two locations where boat fires usually start: the engineroom and the galley.

Water, the natural firefighter, is of no value in extinguishing these fuel conflagrations because it floats the fire and spreads it. Certain chemical powders cover the fire and smother it. Carbon dioxide (CO_2) displaces the air and robs the fire of oxygen needed for burning. Halon, a chlorofluorocarbon liquid/gas, alters the chemistry of oxidation (burning) and makes burning impossible. The powder-containing extinguishers are available in hand-held portable units. The CO_2 and Halon extinguishers are supplied both as portable devices and as fixed engineroom installations. Coast Guard approval is desirable.

The fixed extinguisher installation goes into action either manually or au-

FIRE EXTINGUISHERS

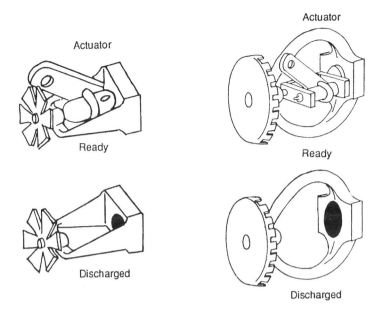

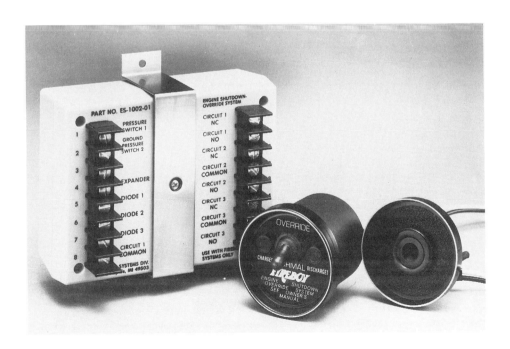

FIRE EXTINGUISHER—The control system, the warning panel, and two discharge jets of a popular fire extinguisher are shown. The "before and after" condition of the jets also is pictured. *(Courtesy Fireboy)*

tomatically. The manual extinguisher requires action by the skipper on a switch or a valve. The automatic extinguisher responds to the rapid rise in temperatrue that melts a fusible link. Obviously, the automatic type is safer because an appreciable period of time may pass before the skipper becomes aware of the fire, and such delay is crucial.

When the engineroom is flooded with extinguishing gas, a gasoline engine will stop because of the worsening of its fuel air ratio. Under the same conditions, a diesel engine may keep running and suck away the beneficial gas before it has completed its work of killing the fire. Hence, engines should be shut down immediately after a fire starts. (Some installations do this automatically.)

A fire needs air in order to burn; hence, the inflow of air should be intercepted as much as possible (for instance, by closing doors). Blowers should be stopped. Professional firefighters say the skipper should be ready to abandon ship if the situation becomes hopeless and endangers life. The smaller the boat, the more likely a fire will cause personal injury.

Installation A fire extinguisher should be mounted *just outside* the space to be protected and *not* inside it. This permits fast escape from the danger area and presents a ready fire extinguisher at a safer position from which to fight the fire—in other words, just outside the engineroom, just outside the galley, just outside *any fire-prone area*. An approved quick-release bracket should be used for mounting the portable cylinders.

Maintenance The purpose of maintenance is to keep the fire extinguishers at the ready. Some extinguishers include a pressure guage calibrated in colored zones of readiness and refill. Some cylinders require weighing to determine their estate of charge. (The Halon cylinder gauge merely verifies sufficient pressure for expelling the contents but not necessarily a full charge of Halon; that must be examined by weighing.)

Replenishment of fire extinguishers is obtained either from local service shops or from the original manufacturer.

Fluxgate Compasses

A long trick at the wheel, steering by compass, emphasizes how continuous observation of a line on the card can tire the eyes. Many helmsmen would prefer a large digital readout of the course. They can have it with the fluxgate compass. Such a choice also provides a bonus by eliminating the compass deviations caused by steel objects nearby on the console.

The comparative freedom of the fluxgate compass from deviationary annoyances is not a built-in feature. Rather, it results from the fact that the magnetic sensor may be placed remotely in whatever section of the boat is most magnetically "clean." An electric cable then connects the sensor with the "repeater" at the console that displays the digital readings. Several repeaters may be connected, in addition—for instance, one on the tower,

FLUXGATE COMPASSES

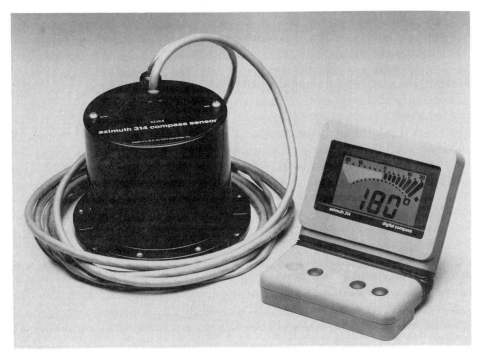

FLUXGATE COMPASSES—The fluxgate compass states its course readings digitally. It has no moving parts, no delicate pivoted card, and is immune to the annoyances of a conventional compass caused by the rolling and pitching of the ship.

The sensor is installed in the most suitable location aboard, while the digital display is placed in the helmsman's line of sight. The two units are connected electrically. *(Courtesy KVH Industries)*

one in the owner's stateroom. (The repeaters, of course, are not affected by surrounding magnetic conditions.)

The display is with liquid crystal screens (LCDs), and may show also a portion of a standard compass card for easier acclimation of the helmsman to the change of display.

The fluxgate compass functions by reason of the effect the Earth's magnetic lines of force have on the inductances in the sensor. The vector sum of these effects is transformed by an electronic circuit into the impulses required to build the digital display. There are no moving parts. The power drawn from the battery is negligible.

Installation Installation of a fluxgate compass and its sensor is easy and obvious. Alignment with the lubber line must be made before final fastening. North–south and east–west screws are provided for compensation.

The fluxgate compass may also be had as a single unit (no remote sensor). This model is affected by nearby magnetic objects, just as a magnetic compass would be (see Compasses).

Fuel Pumps

Automotive engines have generally relied on cam-operated, engine-mounted pumps to force fuel from tank to carburetor. In contrast, marine engines depend on independent electric pumps to transfer the gasoline. These pumps utilize an electrically vibrated diaphragm and are under the control of the ignition switch.

The mechanism is equivalent to an electric buzzer. The short back-and-forth strokes are sufficient to generate the suctions and the compressions needed to move the fuel, and are weak enough to be stopped by the carburetor needle valve when the bowl is full.

Maintenance The fuel pump should get frequent visual inspection. Obviously, a leak here is dangerous.

Repair The fuel pump is non-repairable.

Fuses

A fuse is a one-time, throwaway protector of an electrical circuit. Its method of protection is by melting a connecting link and thereby opening the circuit. Each fuse is rated by the maximum number of amperes it will transmit continuously without "blowing."

The fuses sold for low-voltage marine use are the same as those used for automotive vehicles. They consist of a short length of small-diameter glass tubing sealed at both ends by metal caps. Inside, a link of low-melting-point alloy connects the two caps by being soldered to them. An appropriate base with two clips for the caps holds these fuses. When the link melts, there is no connection between the caps, and the circuit is open. An alternate system is a circuit breaker (see Circuit Breaker).

The fusible link is in series with the load, and all current passes through it. A current beyond the rated value heats the link and melts it. A "blown" fuse is not reusable and is discarded. (A "reusable" fuse is available in which the fusible link may be replaced for reuse.)

A common style of sale of these fuses is five of identical capacity in a small tin box. A "slow-blow" fuse also is available that prevents immediate blow when a motor draws excess current for starting.

Maintenance The maintenance requirement is cleanliness and the prevention of corrosion buildup. The caps and their clips are susceptible to corrosion and the resultant undesirable high-resistance contact. The glass tube makes it easy to spot the dead fuse. (See Trouble Lamps.)

Generator Sets

The manufacturers call it a "generator set," but, more correctly, it is an alternator set because it delivers alternating current. The output of the unit is given in "kilowatts," but, technically, it should be in "kilovolt-amperes," a term that takes into account the power

GENERATOR SETS

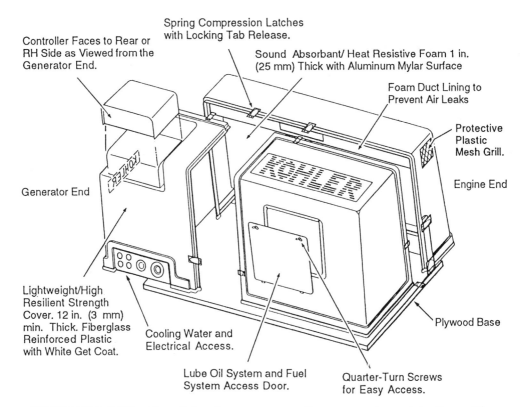

GENERATOR SETS—Close-fitting housings and soundproofing design keep these essential machines quiet. (A popular name for a generator set is "genset") *(Courtesy Kohler)*

factor of the load. (The power factor is a multiplier that is at unity for a lamp-bulb load derates the kilovolt-ampere output by approximately 0.7 when motors are the load.)

A generator set comprises an alternator and a direct-connected gasoline or diesel engine, mounted on a base, plus a control board. The set may be automatic and start in response to the turn-on of anything electrical, or it may require manual starting and stopping. Its terminals supply the standard shore-side voltages of 120/240 to a three-wire system that may have a fourth wire ground. As required for a machine that runs without supervision most of the time, various automatic shutdowns are incorporated.

The alternator part of the generator set has been greatly improved over the years. Earlier machines made use of brushes to take off the power from the rotating windings, and these often became a source of trouble and replacement. The latest machines cleverly dispense with brushes, and handle the output with solid copper connections. Windings are treated with synthetics that protect them from the marine environment.

The output frequency (in hertz) of a

generator set's alternating current is determined by the unit's speed of rotation. Thus, a speed control is an important component. Most controls use some form of spinning weights that open and close the engine throttle in order to maintain the speed rpm constant. The target is as close to 60 hertz as possible, especially if clocks and TVs form part of the load. Voltage is held to close limits by the circuitry.

Generator sets are nosily annoying not only to people aboard but to neighbors as well, and many schemes are used to quiet them. Vibration-absorbing mounts isolate the machine from the structure of the boat that is acting as a sounding board. Covers lined with sound-absorbing materials enclose the generator set (but are easily opened for service). Mufflers cut down on exhaust noise.

The alternator consists of a stator and a rotor, one rotating within the other (see Alternators). It is the well-known procedure of magnetic lines of force being cut by a conductor and generating electricity (see Electricity). The engines may be two-cycle or four-cycle, with up to four cylinders. Engine cooling is by closed-circuit heat exchanger. Extras include an hour meter and other meters, and a shore/ship changeover switch.

Maintenance All generator sets are delivered with complete maintenance and service instructions that should be followed closely.

Troubleshooting Troubleshooting follows two separate logics, one for the alternator and one for the engine.

Switch on, no cranking: Check battery condition and connections. Check circuits to solenoids. Check starter motor.

Cranking but no start: Check fuel shutoff, fuel lines, fuel presence at engine. Check choke (gas engine). Check injectors (diesel). Check for spark (gas). Check for defective automatic shutoff. Check control-panel circuits and relays.

Rpm too high or too low for 60 hertz: Check governor.

Voltage too high or too low: Check voltage regulator circuit. Check for overload.

Repair Voltages around a generator set may be lethal, and persons without direct experience should not attempt repairs.

Grounds

The ground connection of the electronic equipment is perhaps the simplest on the boat, yet it can cause the most widespread trouble when it is not in perfect conductive condition. A loose or corroded ground can make every instrument on the console give incorrect or unsatisfactory readings.

An apt description of a good ground connection is "shiny metal to shiny metal, and tight." The final ground is the one outside the hull, at a location that always stays submerged, and covering several square feet. Claims of extra efficiency by porous metals over plain copper sheet have not been substantiated.

Installation All ground connec-

GROUNDS

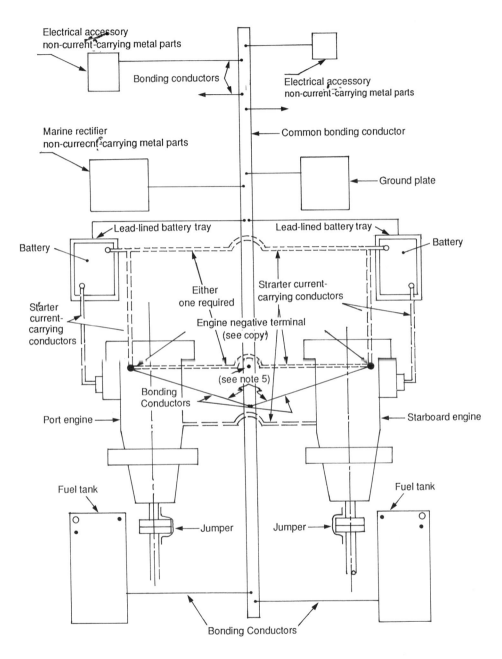

GROUNDS—Shown in this diagram is the American Boat & Yacht Council's suggestion for a bonding system that will hold all onboard metal at ground potential in the interest of safety. *(Courtesy ABYC)*

GROUNDS

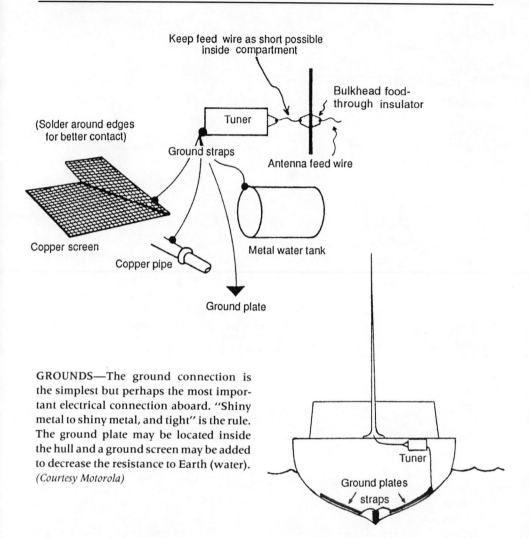

GROUNDS—The ground connection is the simplest but perhaps the most important electrical connection aboard. "Shiny metal to shiny metal, and tight" is the rule. The ground plate may be located inside the hull and a ground screen may be added to decrease the resistance to Earth (water).
(Courtesy Motorola)

tions should be of at least No. 10 copper wire and as short as possible. A long ground wire automatically becomes part of the antenna system; this upsets tuning and makes for skittish operation.

The connection to Earth may be made capacitively with some loss of effectiveness by placing the copper sheet along the inside of the hull. The hull material now acts as the dielectric of a large capacitor. This form of ground gives *no* protection from atmospheric discharges.

A basic, overall grounding system that interconnects all metal installations aboard is recommended. Such grounding is especially protective if a lightning strike occurs nearby, and generates an inductive charge on the boat.

The connections and wiring are made with (preferably) copper strip or with No. 8 copper wire. The effectiveness of this ground system may be checked with a voltohmmeter (see Voltohmmeter).

One test probe of the meter is touched to the main ground line and the other to the metal device in question. The meter should read zero resistance (dead short). Readings between devices should also be zero.

Gyro Compasses

The gyro compass is of interest to the pleasure boatman as a matter of marine education and not (at least for the present) as something he will install and use on his boat. A cost running into the multi thousands is, in itself, a strong reason why the gyro compass is found on nothing smaller than world-class yachts and big ships.

The gyro compass does not make use of magnetism in any manner. It points to true north, and not to magnetic north, as does the standard magnetic compass. It is not affected by local attractions. Most important on big ships, it can automatically supply heading information to other navigational instruments.

The heart of a gyro compass is, quite naturally, a gyroscope. This is a finely balanced flywheel turning at high speed within a gimbaled housing. Such a rotating mass has the unique property of maintaining its orientation in space and keeping its rotational axis parallel to the axis of the Earth. A pendulous weight attached to the gyro housing points to the center of the Earth (gravity) and helps maintain the gyro's spacial attitude.

A gyro compass takes time to get set into its working position. Its motor is switched on hours before getting underway. A gyro compass has several possibilities for error; these are *not* magnetic, but originate in the speed and motions of the ship. These errors are tabulated as errors east and west and are added to or subtracted from the heading.

The main unit of a gyro compass has the bulk approximately of a 10-gallon drum. Course readouts are steady and easy to watch.

Hauling Out

Hauling, to the owner of a 14-foot runabout, means simply calling for the forklift at the marina. In a few minutes his boat will be high and dry on a rack in the shed. To the skipper of a large yacht, hauling is a combination of trouble and expense. Thus, the pros and cons of hauling (taking the boat out of the water for storage or repair) all depend on the size of the boat.

The forklift is the simplest of the hauling devices. In addition there are the marine railway, the Travelift, and the elevator platform. With a marine railway, tracks slope down into the water to a depth greater than the draft of the boat to be hauled. Small railway "cars" pick up the hull and are pulled ashore with the boat by a power cable. The Travelift straddles the boat and picks it up with straps around the hull.

HAULING OUT

The elevator platform is like a huge freight elevator with cars and chocks set up to fit the hull. The platform is raised from the bottom to pick up the waiting hull. Tracks on the raised platform mate with tracks on shore, over which the boat is moved to a repair location.

The experience and skill of the hauling team is the determinant of strain or damage to the hull. There should be enough cars on the railway to cover the length of the hull with correctly spaced chocks. The hauled trim of the boat should be as level as possible. The backbone, the keel, is the vulnerable part of the boat, and carelessness can "break" it.

The Travelift crew puts two or more straps under the hull and locates them at weight points, such as under engines. The tendency these straps have to crush the hull is canceled by crossbars a little longer than the boat is wide, that keep the straps open. The Travelift, with its engine and steering can move all over the yard with its suspended boat. It is well to reduce weight from the boat as much as possible by dumping water tanks and removing heavy items.

The elevator platform is the ideal hauling method for a large boat, but only a few of the larger boatyards are so equipped. While the platform is at shore level, a string of cars is run out on it. A series of chocks is erected on the cars in accordance with a "hauling plan" derived from the yacht designer's drawing. This assures support for the hull at all critical points; the boat is supported almost as evenly as it would be afloat.

If the haulout is to be for a long period, as over the winter, the details of the support should be inspected carefully for strength and placement. The engine room area, with its heavy machinery, needs particular attention. Sailboat masts are unstepped and stored in a protected indoor location. A framework to hold the canvas for snow protection must be constructed (either by yard or by the skipper, depending on agreement and cost). Most large boatyards will supply electricity to large boats when requested, and that may ease problems of work and comfort. Propellers that need repair are removed at this time. Note that the drying-out of a plank-on-frame wooden boat will cause seam leaks, but these are usually self-healing upon reimmersion when the wood swells up again.

The general boatyard custom is to have a fixed charge per foot of length for hauling. This includes taking the vessel out of the water and later putting it back in. It does not include any repair work, although most yards will do a high-pressure water hosedown of the bottom without extra charge. Prior appointments for haulouts are an obvious requirement because of commitments to other customers.

The usual reason for haulouts is bottom painting, as a means of fouling control. The hull material, whether it is wood, fiberglass, or metal, keeps the required work and cost within different ranges. (The least expensive job would be on a fiberglass hull.)

The first crew to take over on a wooden boat is the "bottom gang." With scrapers they remove the vestiges of animal and plant fouling still left after the high-pressure water. They inspect for worm holes and spray them

HAULING OUT

with acetone or copper, to quickly kill the inmates. (Burning ruins wood and is not recommended.) Loose paint is also scraped away.

The first coat of antifouling paint (copper is most popular) now goes on with brush or roller. The optimum time interval between painting and return to the water is stated on the paint can and should be followed.

Each paint manufacturer has series of copper-based antifouling paints with different contents of copper and, consequently, different prices. The top of the line, with the highest copper content, may represent overkill. The most expensive antifouling paint may not provide protection for a longer period than the less costly formulation. Stated succinctly, this may afford some wise economy.

The bottom of the fiberglass boat presents a less difficult problem than the wooden craft just discussed. For one thing, there are no worm holes to find and treat. (Nature has not yet developed a worm that chews fiberglass, but that is no guarantee for the future.) For another, the smooth, glasslike surface of the plastic makes scraping and painting much easier, quicker, and less expensive.

The bottom of the metal hull is a procedure unto itself, and it is advisable to seek a boatyard with like experience. Generally, a barrier coat of special paint will be required to counter electrolysis, and the details are available from the paint manufacturer who usually can recommend a series of paints that work together as a "system."

Many skippers of large yachts live aboard during their stay in the boatyard. This has advantages in supervision and disadvantages in personal comfort. Supervision never hurts with as complex a situation as being hauled. One of the hardships in living aboard for the duration of the yard work is the loss of onboard toilet facilities. Another is the loss of air conditioning, with a water-cooled system. (The good news is that after a couple of experiences, the whole thing becomes quite normal.)

An important safeguard that never should be overlooked occurs immediately after the boat is returned to the water. The yard foreman, flashlight in hand, checks the full length of the bilge for leaks. Such leaks are most likely on a wooden boat, but may occur at through-hull fittings on any hull. The work should not be accepted and the yard bill should not be paid until all leaks are eliminated. In many boatyards, it is customary to make a short trial run, with the foreman aboard, to prove the adequacy of all yard work.

What follows may be called a Guidance List for the age-old tussle between boatyard and boatman:

• Prior to hauling, drive to the boatyard to meet the man in charge and to inspect the facilities. Check the quality of work going on. Familiarize yourself with the best manner of approach with your boat.

• When you bring the boat, have the foreman come aboard, and show him those complaints that are caused by being waterborne. Discuss this and all other matters that will be the responsibility of the yard. Have a hauling plan that shows the required placement of keel blocks and chocks or straps. Drain water tanks, and have as little fuel aboard as possible to reduce weight.

• Make sure every item of work is written clearly in the work order before you sign it. Specify the make and grade of all paint to be used. Insofar as is possible, get at least a "ball park idea" of cost. If you intend to do some work yourself, clear this in advance with the foreman. If the hauling is for winter layup, specify all the winterizing steps to be taken, and set a desired back-in-the-water date.

• Are you authorizing the yard to buy and install new instrumentation? Write down the make and model, also the discount you will receive off the list price and the charges for labor.

• Despite the gauges on fire extinguishers, weighing the units on an accurate scale is still the best method of gauging their readiness for service. Boatyards are regularly visited by the service companies that do this weighing and subsequent filling. Note on the yard order that you want this extinguisher check for your boat.

• Onboard plumbing winterizing should be a number-one thought if the haulout is to be for winter layup. This calls for all water pipes and tanks. There is a preference for filling with antifreeze. Add storage battery care. A difference of opinion exists on whether fuel tanks should be empty or topped up; it is a case of condensation versus sag-producing weight.

• Engine, air conditioning, generator set, etc., all have their owner's manuals. These are "bibles" that should be followed religiously—in the yard or out.

Heads

Translated into landlubber's language, a "head" becomes a toilet. Now that families go boating and a boat no longer is an exclusively male fishing machine, an onboard toilet is considered a bare necessity. Furthermore, federal law and the Coast Guard have come into the picture, and marine toilets are subject to a certain amount of control. The toilets are joined by something comparatively new aboard pleasure boats: holding tanks, (see Holding Tanks). The Coast Guard classifies the equipment as an MSD (Marine Sanitary Device).

The marine toilets of some years ago were small and uncomfortable combinations of a seat and a bowl on a stand that contained a hand pump connected by hose with a through-hull fitting. The pump evacuated the bowl contents directly into the sea and withdrew enough water to rinse the basin. Such simplicity no longer is permitted.

Today's toilets must qualify under one of three Coast Guard classifications: Type I, Type II, or Type III. Each of these three is an active mechanical device. Type I must be able to take human waste and treat it with chemicals and/or maceration (pulverization) to meet minimum/EPA/health standards for discharge into certain restricted waters. Type II must duplicate this, but to a stricter standard. A Type III marine toilet has a choice of the method of waste treatment used, but it may discharge its contents only into a holding tank.

In some waters, the Great Lakes for

HEADS

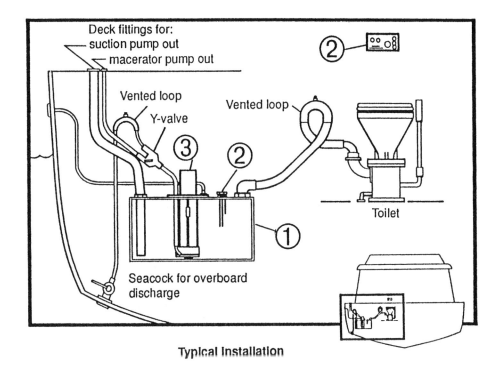

Typical Installation

HEADS—The regulations forbidding overboard discharge have made head installations more difficult than previously. The circuit shown allows a choice of overboard or holding-tank head usage. Overboard discharge is legal more than 3 miles off shore. *(Courtesy Gross Mechanical Labs)*

instance, no overboard discharge is permitted regardless of the type of treatment. Obviously, skippers in those areas have limited choice: either a holding tank or officially sealed toilets.

A solution of sorts could be a portable head. These are carried aboard like a suitcase and are taken ashore for emptying. They are self-contained and require no attachment to the boat. They are not subject to Coast Guard approval.

Boat size also becomes a factor in the correct choice of a head. Vessels over 65 feet in length must equip only with Type III toilets. Smaller boats may choose any of the three types or a portable.

Heads are available for manual and for electric operation. The manual units are much improved over their forebears that required endless pumping. The electric units have simmered down from heavy demands on the battery to sedate demands of as little as 5

HEAT SINKS

amperes. In style, material, and comfort, marine heads have gained much from the improvements in household fixtures.

Installation Onboard toilet installations must be made with a Y-valve. A hose from the toilet connects to the base of the Y. One are of the Y goes to a through-hull fitting. A hose connects the other arm with the holding tank. (See Hose Safety.) Now a swing of the Y-valve lever sets the system up to comply with whatever sanitary regulation confronts the boat.

Maintenance Good maintenance sees to it that all hose clamps are tight and doubled where necessary. A boat flooding via its toilet hull connections is not that rare.

Troubleshooting The recurring problem with marine heads is clogging with foreign matter innocently dumped in by visitors. The recourse is in the owner's manual.

Repair Most manufacturers of heads sell repair kits that contain the likely-to-be-needed parts and full instructions. Work on a head may be messy.

Chinese junks have simplified the response to human needs. A small section of deck extends beyond the stern out over the water. A large hole is centered between two carved footprints. No instructions are needed.

Heat Sinks

Heat sinks are commonly found in electronic construction to protect transistors from their susceptibility to damage from raised temperature. As the name implies, a heat sink accepts unwanted heat and dissipates it to the surroundings. Some heat sinks rely on metal mass; some do the job with radiating fins; some combine both. High-power dissipators even use circulating-cold-water sinks.

Installation The mechanical connection between heat producer and heat dissipater must be close for efficient heat flow. Shiny surfaces are the best radiators, and so cleanliness is

INSTALLATION

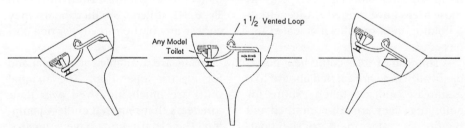

HOLDING TANKS—Heads should be installed at the same level or higher than the holding tanks or the outside waterline. Inlets to holding tanks should always be at the tank top, not on the side. Sparkless sensors may monitor the tanks' contents. *(Courtesy Gross Mechanical Labs)*

worthwhile. (See Soldering Transistors.)

Holding Tanks

Antipollution legislation has turned the boat toilet (head) into a noxious problem. Even the venerable Olde Salt goes beyond the law if he tosses the contents of his bucket into the nation's waters. Human waste generated aboard must be tanked and stored until legal discharge can be made. A holding tank must be provided, either as a permanent installation or as a portable one that may be carried ashore (See Heads).

No lenience is allowed for the fact that the substance handled is the most odious imaginable, and that its putrefaction gives off a dangerous explosive gas called methane (or marsh gas). (A wag has suggested hooking the holding tank to the carburetor.) Holding tanks have exploded, with easily imaginable results.

The capacity of a holding tank must be commensurate with the expected occupancy of the boat. (This is a guesswork dimension, because most people are terrified by a marine toilet and use it only upon sheer necessity.

Holding tanks may be constructed of any noncorrosive material. Fiberglass seems preferred. They may be box-squared in shape or else tailored to fit a given boat space.

Installation If the head is a gravity type, the tank must be lower than the toilet. Plumbing must connect the head (or heads) with the tank. Additional plumbing is needed to provide switching by means of Y-valves. A diaphragm-type pump with large flapper valves should be available if the boat habitually goes three miles offshore, the only legal direct dumping place.

A Y-valve directs the flow from one line into either of two other lines. It is ideal for a holding-tank installation, and two or more will be needed, depending on the number of heads in the system. It should be possible to have a head empty either overboard or into the tank. Likewise, the tank should connect either with the on-deck pump-out fitting or with the through-hull discharge. A "full tank" warning (sparkless) is desirable. Electric pumps designed for holding-tank work also are available; these may be plumbed in permanently to eliminate manual discharge.

The holding tank needs a vent pipe; this prevents lock-up due to either pressure or vacuum. In view of the tank's proclivity for gas and odor, exact location of this vent could be a problem on a small boat. The vent should be in a well-ventilated spot, yet away from people spaces.

Maintenance Regular maintenance can keep the holding tank a reasonably tolerable fellow passenger. The chemicals people have developed a long list of powders, tablets, and liquids especially for the holding-tank situation. Some of these nostrums are added at regular intervals; some are to be put into the head after each use. Some systems are designed to be flushed out completely with seawater—presumably outside the three-mile limit.

HOSE SAFETY

Hose Safety

Clamping a hose to the straight end of piping or tubing is an invitation to future disaster. The trouble stems from the pressure in the system. Despite the tightness of the clamp, the hose will work its way off almost imperceptibly until a complete break results. There is a simple preventive: Bell-mouth the end of the pipe or tube slightly with a ball hammer. The clamp is tightened just aft of the bell.

Hydraulic Steering

Hydraulic systems of control are popular because of the ease of their installation and the smoothness of their action. This is especially true of hydraulic steering systems. Their tubing and hosing may be run around bends without difficulty and in a neat manner; clearances, as for ropes and pulleys, are not required.

The hydraulic-steering system may quickly be converted into "power steering" by adding a power unit run by engine or battery. The installation

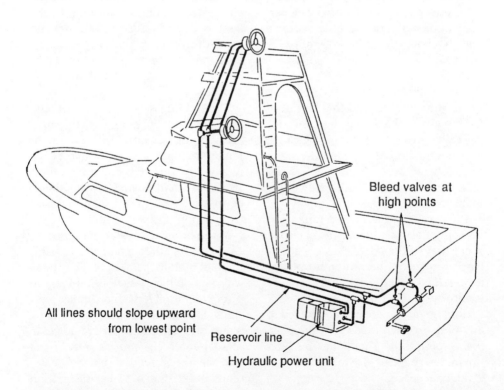

HYDRAULIC-STEERING—Tubing and hosing are run around the boat as needed without difficulty. For "power steering," the power unit is run by the engine or from the battery. (Automotive fluid is used.) *(Courtesy Benmar)*

IGNITION

now becomes a "servo" system that duplicates every movement of the wheel, and provides the effort normally expended by the helmsman. (In non-power, manual systems, the steering wheel assembly contains the pressure-producing pump.)

A bonus from the hydraulic-steering system is the isolation of the steering wheel from the counter-torque of the rudder caused by heavy seas. The helmsman does not have to fight the wheel; the control is always smooth, without the need for additional manual effort.

Maintenance Clearance in hydraulic devices are small and may clog because of incorrect oil and unsatisfactory maintenance. Correct bleeding is important.

Hydrometers

A hydrometer should be aboard every boat that is dependent on lead/acid storage batteries for primary power. This simple instrument quickly gives a reasonably approximate reading of the battery's state of charge and its ability to do work.

The hydrometer consists of a calibrated float inside a transparent tube equipped with a rubber bulb for sucking up samples of the battery electrolyte. (Note that this electrolyte is highly corrosive.) The reading is made by observing the float waterline versus the calibration. Two numbers to remember as a memory jogger are 1,100 and 1,300. Each number is slightly beyond the normal range but serves as a quick check of battery serviceability. (The lower number indicates a dead cell, while the upper number indicates a fully charged cell. Quick-read hydrometers are available that tell battery condition with colored balls that float or sink.

The cells of the battery are tested individually, with three cells to a 6-volt battery and six cells to a 12-volt unit. Specific gravity, the characteristic of the electrolyte measured by the hydrometer, is not the best way to judge the condition of a lead/acid storage battery. Technically superior is testing under load. This is done by simultaneously applying a large ampere load and measuring the voltage drop. Testers that contain a heavy, low-ohmage resistor and a voltmeter are available on the market and are used by battery people. One ingenious manufacturer has combined a battery change-over switch and such a tester for the convenience of boatmen.

Routine maintenance of storage batteries requires regular hydrometer tests plus the replacement of evaporated water. Theoretically, this calls for distilled water, but it is generally agreed that water good enough to drink is good enough for the battery. CAUTION: The gas evolving from a charging battery is explosive. (See Batteries.)

Ignition

The power plants that turn pleasure-boat propellers are internal-combus-

IGNITION

tion engines. This means that the fuel is consumed within the cylinder and not outside it, as in a steam engine. Consequently, some form of ignition must be supplied to set the fuel aflame at the right instant. For gasoline engines, the ignition is electric; for diesel engines, the ignitor is pressure.

Electric ignition may be either low voltage or high voltage. The low-voltage form was known as "make-and-break" because it was similar to touching two current-carrying wires together and "wiping" them apart to make a spark. (One contact "wipes" over the other to clean it before separating and drawing a spark.) Make-and-break was abandoned in the earliest days of engines in favor of high-voltage ignition.

In high-voltage ignition, the spark erupts automatically when the voltage becomes too high for the separation between the contacts in a spark plug. This extreme high voltage is generated by a transformer coloquially called a "spark" coil (see Transformers). It takes the 12 volts of the battery and transforms them to a range of 30,000 to 40,000 volts. (This may sound life-threatening, because the prison electric chair is wired for only 7,000 volts. The difference lies in the fact that the ignition *current* is microscopic, while the current in the chair is lethal.)

The spark in a gasoline engine must arrive exactly within a tiny fraction of a second. This is accomplished by timing—more specifically, by a geared relationshiop with the revolution of the engine crankshaft. Until recently, the gearing caused the opening and closing of two breaker points that controlled the spark. Modern engines have abandoned the breaker points in favor of contactless electronic control that also eliminates condensers, a prolific source of trouble. A stationary pickup coil and a revolving magnet to actuate it take the place of the points.

One difficulty with standard high-voltage ignition is that the voltage builds up at a rate considered slow by electronic rules. As a result, the ignition current can leak around the electrodes of a spark plug and miss a spark. Fully electronic capacitor-discharge ignition overcomes this. It holds back the ignition voltage until it reaches its peak and then dumps it on the spark plug, without the possibility of premature leakage, to ensure a fat spark. (Consider the tank of a toilet. It fills slowly but, when full, dumps its contents in large volume.)

The diesel engine does away with all the details of electric ignition. It ignites its fuel by means of pressure. Cylinder pressure is brought to a value very much higher than that in a gasoline engine. The increased pressure causes ignition temperature to occur within the cylinder. The fuel charge ignites in an excess amount of air for complete combustion. The rising pressure, extreme temperature, fuel ignition sequence is practically instantaneous and takes place in all diesel engines. (See Engines.)

The "timing" of an internal-combustion engine refers to the relationship of the instant of spark to the position of the piston in a gasoline engine, and to the instant of fuel injection to the piston position in a diesel engine. Timing is expressed in degrees before or after top dead center (TDC) of the piston. (Top dead center is highly

IGNITION

critical for engine performance and must be maintained within a degree of the manufacturer's specifications.)

The electric-spark ignition system has many weak points, especially in the marine environment. Old spark plug cables are prone to leakage—and this actually may be seen in the dark. The insides of old distributor caps may be "carbon tracked." This is a carbonizing and breakdown of the plastic surface that diffuses the spark and causes misfiring. Some spark plug cables are made with a high-resistance center to reduce radio interference; vibration may break this central conductor and prevent spark travel.

Many outboard motors generate their own electricity for ignition with a flywheel alternator and therewith eliminate their need for a storage battery. Further simplification is achieved on two-cylinder engines by having two separate spark coils take the place of a distributor.

The equivalent of timing on a diesel engine is the instant at which fuel is squirted into the cylinder. In most diesels, this is accomplished by a central, camshaft-driven pump that feeds the cylinder injectors at a selected piston position. One widely used two-cycle diesel dispenses with the central pump and uses cam-operated individual injectors that build up their own pressure. (The fuel pressure must exceed the high pressure within the cylinder before the fuel can enter.)

Maintenance Electronic ignition (the one without breaker points and condensers) requires little maintenance beyond cleanliness of components, cables, and spark plugs. The timing, once correctly set, does not change.

By contrast, the timing of a breaker-point system does change over a period of use and should be checked at intervals. The change occurs through wear of chain, gear, or the fiber rubbing block on the breaker point arm. In addition, the point contacts should be kept bright and free of burn. A fine-mesh sanding stick, such as the emery boards manicurists use, is a good tool for cleaning point contacts; a touch of grease on it retains sanding dust.

Timing may be checked stroboscopically with a timing light. This is done with the engine running, and it is the most accurate method. Timing of the breaker point system may also be done with a trouble lamp and the engine not running, but this is approximate and disregards the advance mechanism.

Troubleshooting The logical procedure for troubleshooting a balky engine lists the necessary components and then checks to determine whether each is present or absent. Since the immediate concern here is with ignition, this is singled out.

The most direct check for the presence of ignition is to remove a spark plug and, with cable attached, lay it on the engine. If turning the engine over by cranking produces a spark at the plug, the answer is clear: Ignition is not at fault. (Of course, the worst-case scenario, timing trouble, is still possible.)

In the absence of the above-mentioned spark, checking is begun at the battery. If the starter is able to turn the engine normally, the battery charge is within the useful range.

Ignition-circuit continuity may be checked with a simple connection of

INFLATABLES

the trouble lamp (see Trouble Lamps). This light is paralleled across the spark coil primary by connecting it to the two contact screws. Cranking the engine should make the light go on and off rapidly. If the flashing occurs without a resultant spark, the coil may be defective. In the event that flashing does not take place, check back to the breaker points or, rarely, to the breaker-less magnetic pickup coil on the distributor. When condensers are present, they are worthy of suspicion.

Repair Kits are available containing replacement breaker points and condensers and often a small wrench for point adjustment. Distributor caps and cables may also need replacement after long service on a boat.

Inflatables

Inflatables, boats constructed of fabric, that owe their rigidity to the compressed air, may be deflated and folded into a very small space (some even under a plane seat). These are boats of wide usage. They are the boats for the wide-ranging boatman who does not wish to be bothered with a trailer. These boats are chosen for fishing, to act as dinghies that may be stowed out of the way, to be water-skiing towboats. Because inflatables have increased in number so suddenly on the waterways, it is surprising to learn that they have been manufactured for more than 50 years.

The appearance of an inflatable is familiar: a large-diamter, torpedo-shaped air tube at each side, and a connecting structure that forms the floor. A cross board forms the stern and becomes a motor mount. The bow may be brought to a blunt point to cut down water resistance. This basic hull may have refinements such as a steering console, battery and fuel tank enclosures, and bucket seats. (Inflatables are available with fiberglass bottoms for better speed at the cost of less foldability.) Commercial lengths of these craft run approximately from 7 feet to 17 feet.

The construction material is a synthetic fabric, nylon or similar. It is covered, impregnated, and waterproofed, both sides, with an impermeable resin. The developed patterns are brought to correct shape and glued or welded electronically. Reinforcement fabric is overlaid at all seams and attachments. The side air tubes may be divided into compartments by internal bulkheads to assure buoyancy despite accidental puncture.

Inflatables carried aboard for lifesaving in abandon-ship situations are generally more elaborate. They have canvas tops and side curtains for protection from the sun and also carry painters and sea anchors. Many are claimed non-capsizable. (When used commercially, they must meet Coast Guard standards.)

Some inflatables have added touches to please the fisherman. Examples are built-in rod holders, provision for electric bow motors, and self-bailing fixtures in the bottom. (The raised bass seat makes things a bit tippy.)

INFLATABLES

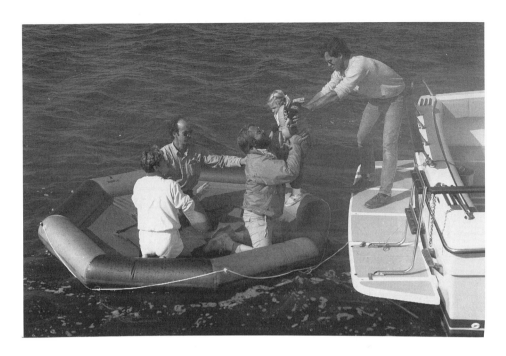

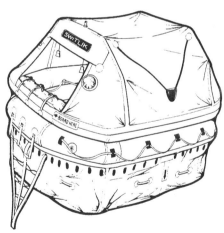 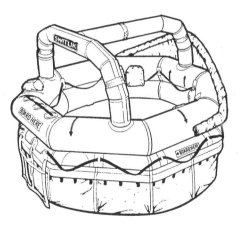

INFLATABLES—Some inflated boats are designed to be used as motor-driven dinghies or even as fast tow-boats for skiers; others are made to be exclusively rescue craft. Two of the latter are pictured. One is a "rescue platform," for use near land where rescue could be imminent. The other shows the construction of a fully protected, inflatable enclosed boat in which offshore survival should be possible for long periods. *(Courtesy Switlik Parachute Co)*

INSURANCE

An inflatable is admittedly clumsy to handle aboard, but its moderate weight makes up for this. A popular carrying location is at the transom on the swim platform. An ingenious carrier device is on the market to simplify stern pickup and launching. Proper towing of an inflatable requires the same care as towing a dinghy.

The high ratio of windage to immersion that characterizes the inflatable explains the difficulty of holding it to a course during a blow. Without wind, the inflatable obeys the helm well.

Maintenance An inflatable should be hosed down after use, and it should be kept out of the sun as much as possible. A simple foot air pump serves for inflation. Cylinders of compressed inert gas may also be used in place of manual effort.

Repair All manufacturers sell kits of material and adhesive with which to make minor repairs. These boats are so tough that the need for repair is not very likely.

Insurance

The knowledgeable, experienced skipper does not cast off from the pier without the mental reassurance that his marine insurance policy is in good shape. The increased boating activity everywhere makes the proper marine policy almost as necessary as fuel.

First, a word of warning: Marine insurance is different from automobile insurance, in both word and deed. A marine insurance specialist is advised—and a good one spots the possible savings in premium.

The insurance protection for a pleasure boat is divided into four areas: Hull insurance, liability insurance, compensation insurance, and medical payments insurance. Hull insurance includes the hull itself plus all machinery required for propulsion. By prior arrangement, fishing equipment may be included in the hull policy. Wear and tear is not compensable. Collision insurance is written as a separate policy.

The liability insurance may be written as "P & I" (protection and liability), and this protects the policyholder against all claims, including any from guests and crew aboard his own vessel. The compensatory clause applies if the vessel employs "paid hands." Medical payments clauses step in when there are medical bills to be settled.

Auto insurance companies have gotten rich on the three little letters "ACV" (actual cash value). The marine policy may be written for the "agreed cash value," and this places the value of the boat beyond argument when the insurance company pays off.

Insurance policies generally restrict the movement of the boat to certain areas during certain seasons. It is wise to obey.

Most insurance companies will allow reasonable policy changes upon request. Competition between the insurance people makes shopping for the lowest premium (with equal benefits) advisable.

Integrating/Interfacing

The skipper who is really into electronic navigation often finds himself at the end of his console space because of the additional equipment required. The solutions may lie in the realms of integrating, interfacing, and redundancy. The bankbook also forms part of the answer.

Integration means that several instruments pool their findings in one console display. Thus depth, speed, temperature, whatever, are shown together, either serially or continuously, on one console face. Space is saved and usually money also. But is this solution as wise as it may appear on the surface? In a certain situation, the loss of three of the four parameters pooled together may be inconsequential, while the fourth (for instance, depth) may be critical.

The money savings brought about by integrating may be much or little, depending largely on the sophistication of the instruments involved. The "works" of a Loran cost more to manufacture than those of a speedometer. (Serial digital display may save money in integration by requiring only one active viewing screen.)

Interfacing allows the units in a coordinated electronic installation to "talk" with one another. The Loran may supply the GPS (Global Positioning System; see Satellite Navigation Systems) with precise ground data; the speedometer may supply the numbers to permit an accurate "time to next waypoint" readout.

Redundancy, the duplication of active instruments, is the safest procedure for passagemakers—and obviously also the most expensive, and the most avid user of console space.

Note that the "conversation" between instruments takes place at higher and higher frequencies as the operation becomes more and more sophisticated. The necessary connectors and coaxial cables for the interconnections must be chosen to specifications; they must be operative at the extremely high frequencies in vogue today. A proper high-grade capacitor properly connected at the origin of radio interference will absorb and eliminate trouble.

Inverters

The *in*verter performs a function opposite to that of the *con*verter. The converter supplies battery current from an alternating-current source, while the inverter changes battery current into alternating current (see Electricity). Thus, without any rotating machinery, small household AC appliances may be operated aboard from the boat storage battery (the emphasis is on 'small'); see Batteries.

The amount of current taken from the battery is the reason for the restriction on appliance size. To illustrate this, consider an electric kitchen mixer that draws 1 ampere at 120 volts AC. Assuming a theoretically perfect circuit with no transformation losses (and

Nature does not allow that), the current drawn from the battery would have to be 10 amperes. Consequently, as a rule of thumb, figure battery current to be *more* than ten times the appliance current. The voltage ratio, input to output, is 1 to 10.

Modern inverters have abandoned the old-time vibrating reed as the source of the AC frequency. A solid-state oscillator/power amplifier set to 60 hertz has been substituted; there are no moving parts. Some inverters feature "automatic load sensing"; this turns the inverter on to pick up the boat's AC load whenever pier power fails. Voltmeters and ammeters also are available to monitor inverter performance (see Ammeters, Voltmeters)

Installation The marine inverter is well insulated against the environment, but it should be protected against spray.

Maintenance While the inverter is in operation, it is wise to check frequently for overheating. To do this, carefully touch the inverter with a wetted finger; the inverter should not rise in temperature beyond decidedly warm.

Jet Drives

A jet drive provides motive power and direction for a boat without the use of propeller, rudder, or reverse gear. It consists of a steerable, reversible stern jet fed by an engine-driven, high-volume, high-pressure water pump.

The jet drive is a reactive device that obeys Nature's law that every action has an equal and opposite reaction. The water ejected rearward by the jet is the action, and the resulting forward thrust of the boat is the reaction (see Propellers). A baffle on the jet may be moved to eject the water forward and provides reverse. Steering is accomplished by swinging the jet in a horizontal plane to the desired direction.

The jet drive has no rotating mass of metal, such as a propeller and shaft, and is practically free of inertia, making instantaneous changes of speed possible. Headway may be killed quickly by swinging the jet into reverse (as jet planes do).

Installation A through-hull fitting, in the bottom amidships, supplies water to the pump; a grating protects against fouling ingestion. Obviously, the intake location must remain immersed regardless of trim or speed. The pump is below the waterline and needs no suction ability; hence, a centrifugal type is eminently suited. (It takes much power to pump water, and the pump always appears small compared to the engine.)

Grounding is bad for any hull, but the location of the intake makes grounding especially disastrous for a jet drive.

Knotmeters

Unlike automobile speed, which always refers to the coverage of a finite distance over the ground, boat speed may be either over the ground or

KNOTMETERS

through the water and must be identified. With boat speed, the same run could yield two widely disparate figures.

When assessing the performance of a boat, the important parameter is speed through the water. When piloting, speed over the ground becomes the critical figure. Different methods of measurement are required to produce the two dissimilar results.

The "knot" is the unit for nautical speed statements. A boat is at a speed of one knot when it traverses one nautical mile in one hour. (The statute mile is 5,280 feet. The nautical mile is 6,076 feet.)

Note that this is *not* "knots per hour," a common error. As students of physics will realize, knots per hour becomes an acceleration instead of a velocity. At a knots-per-hour rate, the boat soon would be traveling with the speed of a projectile.

A knotmeter may sense speed hydraulically, mechanically, electronically, or with a Doppler procedure. The simplest is the hydraulic, and hence it is the lowest in cost and the most popular. The most accurate and the most costly is the Doppler, found on large commercial vessels. The Doppler method alone is able to measure speed over the ground directly.

The sensor for the hydraulic system is the Pitot (pronounced "pee-toe") tube, long used in aviation. An open-ended tube points ahead into the boat's slip stream and also has a counter opening. The pressures developed are fed by plastic tubing to a sensitive pressure gauge calibrated in knots or in miles per hour.

A different form of sensor feeds information to the mechanical/electronic speedometers (knotmeters). This sensor is a small paddle wheel fitted into the hull. The paddle contains a magnet that generates a pulse in a pickup coil at each revolution. These pulses are fed to the console indicator by a wire connection. The indicator counts the number of pulses per unit of time, or measures the frequency, and reduces this to a reading on a dial calibrated in knots, or in miles per hour. The reading is speed through the water and must be corrected for wind and current if it is to be used in a position-finding problem.

Installation The location of the speed sensor has a bearing on the accuracy of the readings. Where a boundary layer of water travels with the hull, a sensor's reaction would be ambiguous and unreliable. Areas on a planing hull that rise out of the water at speed obviously are taboo for a sensor.

Troubleshooting The most accurate, and the simplest, method of checking the accuracy of a boat speedometer is with a radar gun. These are professionably available, and inquiry may help you find one.

The common manner of checking speedometers is by running a measured mile. A number of such miles are shown on charts and have readily identifiable markers.

The test should be made on a day as devoid of wind and current as possible. A stopwatch or a good watch with second hand is used for timing. Immediately on finishing a run, it is repeated in the opposite direction, and the times

LEAD LINES

are averaged. (Note whether the mile is statute or nautical.)

Lead Lines

An ingenious, easily constructed lead line is made with fishing line (preferably linen) and a number of 1-inch-diameter cork ball floats, plus a 6-ounce (or heavier) sinker. This lead line is handy to use and trustworthy in its readings because the line remains vertical from bottom to waterline.

The cork balls are threaded onto the line at exactly 1-foot intervals starting with the bottom of the sinker. Small wooden pegs are cut and are used to jam each ball at its properly spaced position on the line. A red-painted ball is pegged to the line at a distance from the tip of the sinker exactly equal to the minimum depth of water required by the boat.

A discarded electric-wire spool is a good way to store this lead line between times of usage.

Reading the depth is aided by marking ball No. 5, ball No. 10, etc.

How long to make the lead line is determined by the depths of the waters normally cruised.

Life Rails

The decks of pleasure boats provide precarious footing at best, and life rails and lifelines are required safety equipment. The installations on sailboats are usually sturdier than those on powerboats, and with good reason: Heavy weather can mean a crew will be on deck working the sails and relying on the lifelines to prevent going overboard. Under the same storm conditions, powerboat crews stay below.

The standard sailboat lifeline consists of a series of stanchions threaded by stranded stainless-steel wire. The line is kept taut by turnbuckles. The open construction makes it easy for a harnessed person to hook himself on. A wire at the top and a wire at mid-height is the usual design, and such spacing is considered adequate.

At one time, powerboat rails were chosen for their decorative value, with little thought for practical safety. The rails were low and, instead of preventing a fall overboard, actually helped pitch a person over. Modern design specifies full-height life rails for powerboats, generally with solid railing in place of the stainless stranded wire.

The popularity of anchor pulpits has made an opening in the lifeline at the bow necessary. In one scheme, the line stops at each side of the pulpit; in another, the line follows the contour of the pulpit and protects the person making the anchor.

Installation The stanchions must be through-bolted with a backing plate (see Cleats). It is not unusual for a crew member to lose his footing and to be hurled broadside into the lifeline. Obviously, the lifeline installation must survive much stress without hint of failure.

Maintenance Recommended maintenance is to periodically check the tightness of the through-bolts holding the stanchions, and take up slack with the turnbuckles.

Lightning Rods

Lightning storms are occurring continuously around the Earth, yet the possibility is small that a given boat will take a direct strike during its lifetime. Nevertheless, a prudent skipper will protect his vessel, just on the off chance that lightning will strike—all the more, because protective procedure is not difficult.

The magnitude of lightning power taxes the imagination. Millions of volts, millions of amperes, trillions of watts. Were the flash continuous, it would outrival all the utility stations of the world combined. But a lightning flash lasts only a few millionths of one second, and the unleashed power is mammoth enough to cause the familiar destruction in that instant of time.

The birthplace of the electricity is the cumulo-nimbus cloud known as a thunderhead, and the method of generation is thought to be friction within a friendly ambiance of temperature, pressure, and moisture. Millions of small charges add up to a difference of potential between positive and negative great enough to break down the intervening air. The results are flashovers, sometimes to another cloud, often to the earth. The earth flashes are preceded by thin, trial discharges that ionize the path for the main, heavy, damaging, full-power strike.

The current in the flash heats the air through which it bores so rapidly that the instant expansion and collapse are heard as thunder. The temperatures reach the thousands of degrees. The shock waves of sound travel outward and are heard nearby as a crack and farther away as a rumble.

The increasing static on an AM radio is an excellent forewarning of lightning.

The damage caused by lightning is due to the enormous electric currents that are caused to flow. First of all, there is heat, a familiar condition when any current overcomes the resistance in any conductor. With lightning the heat is so instantaneous and so great that even heavy conductors simply melt and start fires. The flash burns a long "hole" in the air through which it passes, and when this collapses shock waves are formed that do blast damage.

Electrical problems may prove to be the most disrupting and the costliest heritage of a lightning strike. The heavy current generates an intense magnetic field that acts like the primary of a huge transformer. All nearby conductive objects become secondaries and receive destructive induced currents. Radios and navigational electronics burn out, and the compass goes wild and needs a new deviation table.

The foregoing is the normal progression of events. Luckily, much of the trouble may be prevented with a correct anti-lightning installation.

Installation Electricity, lightning included, always seeks the best and shortest path to ground. The mast of a boat on a broad expanse of flat water is such a path—hence, the lightning rod at the tip of the mast. Should the end of the rod be pointed or a small ball? Both are effective, depending on the nature of the electric field surrounding them. (The sharp point is better at discharging the field and preventing a strike.)

The other terminus of the lightning path is the copper ground plate on the bottom of the hull. (Claims that a "porous" metal block makes a more effective ground have not been proved by measurement.) The connection between mast tip and ground plate should be copper wire no less than B&S No. 4. Sharp turns in direction and tight bends should be avoided. Every metal mass aboard should have its own No. 4 to the ground-plate connection, brought through the hull to bleed off induced currents. The idea is to have everything aboard at the same potential to avoid flashes from one metal mass to another. An easier and neater installation may be possible with B&S No. 20 copper strip about 1½ inches wide instead of the No. 4 wire.

It is believed that a correctly installed anti-lightning system provides a "cone of protection" for the boat. The apex of this cone is the lightning rod, and from there down the invisible boundary is at a 60-degree angle. With a reasonable height of mast, most medium-sized boats would be covered; sailboats surely would be.

It has been suggested that sailboats with stainless-steel standing rigging use it for the down lead from the lightning rod. This is not recommended, because of the high electrical resistance of the stainless.

Troubleshooting A jury rig is suggested for boats not equipped with lightning rods. Fasten a heavy copper wire to a long, heavy, wooden boathook so that the bared copper projects like a lightning rod. The other end of the wire is fastened to a copper plate immersed overboard.

At the warning of a storm, bind the boathook as high to the mast as possible. CAUTION: Stay as far away from this rig as possible during the lightning storm.

Loran-C

Loran-C pinpoints a location at sea by measuring the difference in times of arrival of pairs of radio signals. The signals are sent by groups of transmitters called "chains," each consisting of a master M, a secondary W, a secondary X, a secondary Y, and a secondary Z. The time difference (TD) of arrival from M and W is called TDW, from M and X it is TDX, from Y it is TDY, and from Z it is TDZ. The TDs are referred to a proper chart with labeled curves. Each curve is a line of position (LOP), and where two LOPs cross, the result is a fix.

The chains are identified by their Group Repetition Interval (GRI). The GRI is the total time in microseconds between the start of a master transmission and the start of the following master transmission; it includes sufficient time for all the secondaries to transmit. For instance, the East Coast chain has an interval of 99,300 microseconds. (The final zero is dropped for convenience, and the correct listing is 9,930.) As a further example, the GRI of the North Atlantic chain is 7,930.

LORAN-C

The GRI is the number to which the Loran-C is tuned. The instrument recognizes the chain by that time interval and rejects other chains that differ from it. Once the GRI is fed into the Loran-C of today, there is nothing further for the operator to do except wait a minute or two for a reading. This reading may be in TDs for referral to a specially Loran-marked chart, or it may be in latitude and longitude for use with a standard chart.

The radio transmissions to a Loran-C consist of pulses. The master sends eight pulses each separated by 1,000 microseconds and adds a ninth separated by 2,000 microseconds. (This is for recognition.) Each secondary sends eight pulses separated by 1,000 microseconds. A "secondary coding delay" controls the starting time of each secondary transmission.

The Loran-C system depends upon the ability to measure the passage of time in millionths of one second, but this presents no problem because the electronic circuits can do this accurately. A loss in accuracy may occur from causes connected with the travel of radio waves, especially waves as low in frequency and as extended in length as Loran-C emissions (100 kilohertz and 3,000 meters).

The ultra-long Loran-C waves suffer some diffraction when moving from land to water and vice versa, and the effects of this must be factored out to preserve accuracy. This correction is called the Additional Secondaryphase Factor (ASF). Present-day Loran-C instruments compensate automatically. Compensation for magnetic variation also is automatic.

The radio noise level about the antenna, the signal-to-noise ratio (SNR), plays an important part in the functioning of the Loran-C. When the signal does not rise clearly above the noise level, and thus allow the receiver to latch onto it precisely, it takes longer for the Loran-C to settle down to a reading. Notch filters are adjusted to eliminate interfering transmissions. (A notch filter is an electronic trap into which an offending signal discharges its energy and becomes harmless.) Onboard sources of electrical noise include all electric devices and even fluorescent lights.

Because the Loran-C takes minutes to complete its calculations, the following caution is necessary when setting a waypoint while underway: The boat should remain stationary at the waypoint until the Loran-C settles down to a good reading. Failure to follow this caution results in memorized waypoints that may be in error by considerable distances.

Loran-C readouts use liquid crystal display screens (LCDs) that are reasonably readable even in sunlight. Telephone-type digital buttons accept the GRI number that selects the chosen chain.

Installation The standard Loran-C antenna is a plain 8-foot whip devoid of internal coils or capacitors. It is mounted on a metal box that contains a preamplifier. A cable takes the amplified signal to the Loran-C and also supplies the direct current for the transistor preamplifier.

The antenna should be located where it has a clear "view," away from all metal objects that could reradiate spurious, misleading signals. A good ground to the preamplifier box is es-

LUBRICATING OILS

sential; it should lead directly to the ship's main ground and consist of copper tape or heavy copper wire (see Grounds).

Maintenance An overall check of a Loran-C installation is conveniently made at the home pier. The exact location is known, both by TDs and by latitude/longitude, and thus may be used to check the accuracy of the readings. A test of onboard electrical noise may also be made here easily.

The Loran-C is fired up with everything else turned off, and its operation is closely observed. Engines, bilge pumps, TVs, whatever, are then turned on individually, with particular attention paid to any degrading of Loran-C performance. A noticeable decline indicates a need for filters, usually capacitors, to take out unwanted radio frequencies. A truly bad SNR will elicit an automatic warning. (SNR denotes "signal noise ratio," a measure of signal quality.)

The ground connection at the antenna preamplifier box is critical. It should be checked frequently for corrosion. (See Antennas and Grounds.)

Lubricating Oils

Without lubricating oil, mechanical devices could not exist. Metal moving on metal without an intermediate protective lubricant would quickly grind itself to failure. In a properly lubricated situation, the moving metals do not touch each other but are microscopically separated by a lube film.

In the pleasure-boat field there are several categories of demand for lubrication. Inboard engines, outboard engines (both gasoline and diesel), sterndrives, transmissions, and reverse gears all have their individual appetites for manufacturer-recommended lubrication. Each lube is recognized by its commonly known grade and by its technical specifications. Often, the name of the producing company is an important factor in the choice.

Modern oils are expected to do more than lubricate. Among the required extra features are: the ability to keep the engine internally clean, the power to disperse contaminants, and the ability to place a minimal load on the filters to assure extended filter life. Furthermore, the lube should be a good conveyor of heat, be zinc-free, and be neutral in acidity.

The severity of service the oil can endure is rated by the industry with a two-letter code. Examples are: CA, CB, CC, CD, SB, SC, SD, SE, SF, in ascending order. Diesel-engine service is considered to be tougher than gasoline-engine service, and the ratings make that distinction.

The "specs" on a lubricating oil would include the viscosity, the pour point, the flash point, the ash content, and the zinc content. The ash content should be at a minimum for oils intended for use in two-cycle engines that need mixing of oil and gasoline. (The tendency to reduce the percentage of oil added to gasoline for two-cycle engines increases the severity on the oil of this service.)

The industry has some extreme tests for the oils they produce. One of these runs a heavily loaded engine under less than optimum conditions for 24 hours. No preignition may occur while the engine is running. An inspection after shutdown may reveal no signs of scoring or scuffing. No deposits are allowed to have accumulated.

The heavier oils for transmissions and gearboxes are judged as critically. (A special oil for air-conditioning and refrigeration systems is wax-free. This is necessary because the oil in the air-conditioning system flows with the refrigerant, and the wax would quickly harden and stop operation.) Gear oils are fortified against the high pressures generated where gear teeth mesh.

Typical specifications for an outboard-engine oil (two-cycle) are as follows:

Viscosity at 100°F	137
Viscosity at 210°F	44
Viscosity index	57
Flash point (°F)	134
Pour point (°F)	−35

Maneuvering Boards

While running in open water, the skipper sees a vessel far off to starboard that is apparently on a course converging with his own. Does this portend a hazardous situation in the making? Under the Rules of the Road, the other boat would have the right of way. Should our skipper change course and prepare to cross astern? Assuming the present situation continues unchanged, what will be the "closest point of approach" (CPA)?

The answer to the foregoing is found quickly by plotting, and the most convenient method is with a "maneuvering board." A maneuvering board is a printed sheet with polar coordinates and distance scales. It is supplied in pads under the official number HO-2665-10. The two parameters required for the maneuvering-board plot are angle in degrees and distance in miles. Both may be taken directly from a radar scope.

For instance, if the skipper's first reading was 4 miles and 94 degrees, those figures would be entered on the maneuvering board. If five minutes later the reading shifted to 3 miles and 90 degrees, those figures would be placed on the board. After an additional five minutes a third radar reading would be made. If the reading was 2 miles and 80 degrees, that point would be marked and a total of three points of intersection would be in place on the manuevering board.

A line drawn through these particular points would be a straight line showing that the other boat is maintaining its speed. Since this line passes well ahead of the skipper; there is no danger of collision. The actual distance to the closest point of approach (CPA) is obtained by drawing a perpendicular from the board center to the line of approach. Here it would be two miles.

The various scales printed on the maneuvering board present quick solutions to time-speed-distance problems.

An important caution supersedes all plotting: If successive sightings of the other boat remain the same, and if the separating distance is decreasing, collision is imminent. *Change course.*

Mildew

Mildew is a prime nuisance on boats that have enclosed spaces that are not fully ventilated. Mildew is a mold that thrives in locations damp, warm, and not open to free air circulation. The mold is in the air everywhere in unknown trillions.

The first visible indication of mildew damage appears as a light stain. The damage is done because the mold feeds on the surface that attracted it. If this happens to be the waxy film on a polished panel, the result can easily be imagined. (The mold will not "eat" synthetics but will attack almost everything else.)

The only favorable aspect of mildew is the ease with which it may be removed when it has not been allowed to get too strong a foothold—in other words, when it is detected early on. Soap and water are effective, especially if a shot of bleach is added. A good detergent works even better. Rubbing the stain with a rag moistened in detergent is effective for clothing.

The market offers many sprays and liquids with which to fight mildew. some of these are cleaners, some are preventives. A good rule is to try the procedure first in a hidden corner.

The sun is an excellent "for-free" mildew killer. It will also kill the molds that have not yet visibly sprouted. If what ever is mildewy can be left in the sun, the war is half won.

The general rule for mildew prevention aboard is to ensure good ventilation. Louvers on all enclosed spaces, drawers left open, closets heated by low-wattage electric light bulbs (CAREFUL) or warning rods—all of these help to ward off mildew. Paradichlorobenzene (moth crystals) sprinkled in drawers is also helpful. (Keep it away from plastic.)

Navigation Lights

Navigation lights (running lights) are carried by pleasure boats in accordance with Coast Guard Regulations. These "CG Regs" specify the color and luminescence of the lights, their legal locations aboard the boat, and the distances over which they must be visible under normal conditions. The angle over which each light projects its beam is closely held to by its manufacturer.

A casual inspection of boat lights in a pleasure-boat harbor reveals two facts: (1) Location and color and angle are in close agreement with the CG Regs. (2) The visibility specification is widely ignored. This is as true of the gilt-edged vessel as of her poorer sisters. The reason for the lack of conformity is a basic one: The low-voltage, low-amperage electric bulbs cannot draw enough power to generate light able to travel miles.

The housing of these lights is brass, for low corrosion, with the transparent portion either glass or plastic in the familiar Fresnel shape (external surrounding ridge). Light-exit openings are either 112.5 degrees for side lights, 135 degrees for stern lights, 225 degrees for masthead lights, and 360 degrees for anchor lights. Colors are red for a port light, green for a starboard light, and white for lights in other lo-

NAVIGATION LIGHTS

Vessel under 12 meters in length

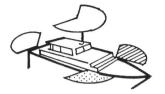

White masthead light visible 2 miles
Side lights or combination light visible 1 mile
Stern light or all-round light visible 2 miles

or

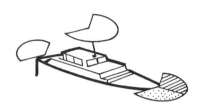

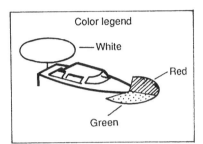

Color legend
— White
Red
Green

or

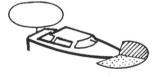

Vessel 12 to less than 20 meters in length

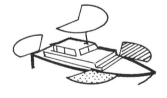   or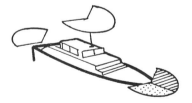

Masthead visible 3 miles   Combination sidelight or sidelight visible 2 mile
Sternlight visible 2 miles

Courtesy American Boat & Yacht Council

NAVIGATION LIGHTS—The internal construction of a masthead light is shown. *(Courtesy Guest)*

115

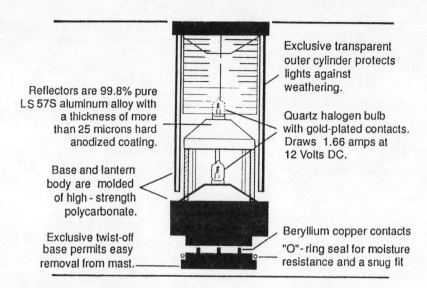

Reflectors are 99.8% pure LS 57S aluminum alloy with a thickness of more than 25 microns hard anodized coating.

Base and lantern body are molded of high-strength polycarbonate.

Exclusive twist-off base permits easy removal from mast.

Exclusive transparent outer cylinder protects lights against weathering.

Quartz halogen bulb with gold-plated contacts. Draws 1.66 amps at 12 Volts DC.

Beryllium copper contacts "O"-ring seal for moisture resistance and a snug fit

NAVIGATION LIGHTS—These illustrations show the legal running lights for vessels in three categories underway. Depicted are (1) power-driven vessels, (2) sailing vessels, and (3) sailing vessels under power. Anchor lighting is not shown but consists of a 360-degree white light at the top of the mast.

Vessel Under Sail and Power or Sailboat Under Power Alone Optional*

Vessels Under 20 Meters

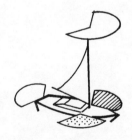   or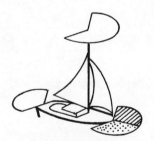

Ranges

Under 12 meters in length

Masthead - 2 miles
Side lights - 1 miles
Stern light - 2 miles

12 meters to less than 20 meters in length

Masthead - 3 miles
Side lights - 2 miles
Stern light - 2 miles

*Note: A vessel under sail and power, or a sailboat (auxiliary) under power alone, for purpose of light configurations is considered a power driven vessel when underway.

Courtesy American Boat & Yacht Council

NAVIGATION LIGHTS

Sailing Vessels Underway

Sailing Vessels Under 12 Meters in Length-Under Sail Alone

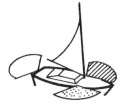 or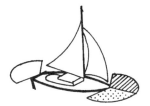

Combination side light or
side lights
visible 1 mile

Stern light visible 2 miles

Tri-color light ranges as
above red & green 1 mile
white sector 2 miles

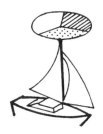

Sailing Vessels from 12 Meters to Under 20 meters in Length - Under Sail Alone

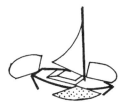 or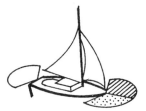

Combination side light or
side lights
visible 2 miles

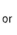 or

Stern light visible 2 miles

Tri-color light ranges as
above red & green 2 miles
white sector 2 miles

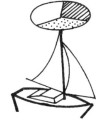

Courtesy American Boat & Yacht Council

NAVIGATION MARKERS

cations. Small boats are permitted to combine red and green in one lamp for use at the bow. The required intensity of the lights is specified on the basis of boat size and light position and ranges from visibility at 2 miles (small boat) to 6 miles. Note the underway illustrations for power, sail, and sail plus power.

Maintenance Lights should be kept clean and should be visually inspected often enough to ensure their functioning when required (nights and bad weather). The constant exposure to weather makes life difficult for contacts such as those on bulb bases. Frequent cleaning of these contacts with fine abrasive paper is recommended.

Navigation Markers

A vast system of buoys, lights, beacons, and other so-called "markers" connects the waters of the United States and enables an experienced skipper to cruise from place to place in safety. The experience needed to follow the system is only moderate and can be acquired easily. As is to be expected, nighttime passages are made a bit more difficult by the confusing lights from shore (see Night Boating), but, here again, a few cautious trials bring good results.

Simple rules of shape and color translate the message conveyed by each navigation marker into the "lateral system" or into the "cardinal system." The lateral system directs a boat *laterally* to port or to starboard of a marker. In the cardinal system, the boat is directed *cardinally* to a compass quadrant of the marker. In general, the lateral system includes all markers on "navigable" waters, while the cardinal system functions for Western rivers.

Note that the designation "navigable water" has no reference to size or depth. A navigable water is one that gives access to another state or to a foreign country. The U.S. Coast Guard controls and services about 40,000 markers on navigable waters. Waters within the boundaries of a state are under the jurisdiction of that state, but markers have been kept to a common standard by agreement.

Markers attain their high value as aids to navigation because they are carefully identified on charts. This allows a skipper to correlate what he sees and what the chart details—in other words, to "fix" his position. Immediate dangers are thereby brought to his attention.

Buoys are a widely used form of navigation marker. When the above-water portion is cylindrical, the buoy is called a "can"; when conical, the buoy is called a "nun." Cans are painted green (formerly black) and nuns are painted red. Some course instructions may involve only one form of marker, as, for instance, "red right returning" when returning from the "sea," keep red markers on the starboard side.

Buoys follow many patterns, but all are easily identified as cans or nuns. Buoys may or may not carry additional warning devices such as bells, horns, or lights. All these additions are identified on charts and are welcome steering aids in bad weather. Unfortunately, the bells and whistles and other

NAVIGATION MARKERS

attention-getting devices depend on rough water for operation, and a calm, foggy day leaves them silent. (The Coast Guard is planning a switch to electrically operated buoys.)

Buoys are anchored to the bottom, and this gives them an aura of accuracy that often they do not deserve. The local conditions may require considerable scope in the anchoring chain, causing a large circle of position of the buoy; this may be large enough to lead to navigational errors. Also, despite a heavy concrete "sinker," the buoy may have been moved by storm or by collision with a vessel. The good judgment of a skipper has no substitute here.

A buoy may serve two waters simultaneously. The Indian River and the Intracoastal Waterway form a case in point. These buoys serve the Indian River in the normal manner and then, by adding a yellow symbol, give the skipper ICW information as well. A yellow square causes the buoy to be considered an ICW can, while a yellow triangle makes the buoy an ICW nun.

The heavy, steel construction of buoys makes them good reflectors of radar signals and leads to clear blips on boat radar screens. In the most modern equipment, the blip will identify the buoy.

Navigation markers may be equipped with lights for clearer, more positive identification under all conditions. The addition of light is clearly shown on the chart. This light may be steady (rare); or it may flash slowly or quickly, or "occult." The light pattern takes a given number of seconds to complete (2½, 4, or 6 seconds), and this becomes another method of identification on the chart.

Unlike buoys, beacons are built directly into the ground and eliminate the error of scope. A day beacon may be little more than a sign (square green or triangular red) to verify the course for the helmsman. The Morse code is a common form of identification of lights. For example, a short flash followed by a long flash conveys the letter A.

The lights on navigation markers are either green (for cans) or red (for nuns), and beacons are painted red or green accordingly. Special-purpose non-directional markers may be yellow with yellow light.

Be on the lookout for special-purpose buoys and day beacons. Green and red horizontally banded buoys mark channel junctions and hazards that may be passed on either side, depending on instructions. With the top band green (as seen from the helm), pass with the marker to port; with the top band red, pass with the marker to starboard. Red and white vertically striped markers (buoys) are mid-channel separators and should be passed on either side close aboard, without regard to can or nun shape.

A quick example will fix the difference for the skipper between the lateral and the cardinal systems: A wreck in the *lateral* scheme (navigable waters) requires a marker directly above it; a *cardinal* warning for that wreck (Western rivers) would direct traffic away from it by compass to denote a safe area.

The Coast Guard Regulations make allowance for private aids to navigation. A club or a well-known restaurant may mark its entrance channel.

NIGHT BOATING

The private markers are allowed wide latitude in design and become the legal responsibility of the people that placed them.

All navigation markers are protected by law. It is illegal to damage a marker, to tie up to it, to obstruct it from view. All collisions with a marker must be reported to the Coast Guard.

Night Boating

Without personal experience, it is hard to believe that a boating area, totally familiar by day, can be unrecognizable at night. Lights ashore are the culprit. Markers fade into the general pattern. Automobile tail lights suddenly become running lights of ghost ships. The loom of general sky lighting ashore hinders the eyes watching on the water.

The human eye can accommodate to a wide range of light colors and intensities, but, except in the very young, it is a comparatively slow process. Once the helmsman's eyes are comfortable with the red-lighted compass, they should be protected from white light. Even a quick beam from a flashlight can destroy his accommodation to the low red and leave him "blind" for many minutes.

Instrument lights may become a problem. Despite its low candlepower, the bulb in a console meter can light up the wheel area to look like Broadway. A rheostat (dimmer) should be in series with all instrument lights to allow the man on watch to set his own comfort level.

Night practice in a familiar area is highly recommended so that proper instrument light intensity can be ascertained and night navigation can become second nature. If there is any danger from rocks or shoals in the practice area, their locations should be memorized and used as a constant check on boat position. Needless to say, practice runs should be "dead slow" until a degree of proficiency is reached.

Traditionally, at night the navigation desk has been lit by a red light. However, recent tests have convinced the U.S. Navy that a variable-intensity white light is best. The tests indicate that when the white light is set at the same intensity as a red light, not only is the chart—especially the red markings—more clearly seen, but also that full night vision is restored just as swiftly after the light is extinguished.

Outboard Motors

The outboard motor was born as a clumsy, heavy appendage for the rowboat transom; it could barely generate 1 horsepower but nevertheless eliminated rowing. The outboard has developed into today's finely tuned machine whose horsepower can top 300. It has a respectable ratio of weight to power and an enviable record of reliability.

The clever idea that underlies outboard-motor design is to support the engine with its crankshaft vertical instead of (the usual) horizontal. This concept, which allows 90-degree internal gearing and a horizontal propeller

OUTBOARD MOTORS

shaft, set a style and shape universally followed by all manufacturers. (The stern-drive also uses 90-degree gearing in its system; see Stern-Drives.) Depending upon horsepower, the number of cylinders in the engines ranges from one to eight. Block style is in-line or vee. Starting is by hand (see Rope Starters) or by battery (see Starters). Engine ignition may be either by magneto, by coil (either with or without breaker points), or by capacitor discharge (see Ignition).

Discharging the engine exhaust through the propeller hub has become standard and offers a bonus in efficiency: The action of the prop creates a suction that lowers the unwanted back pressure in the exhaust pipe that wastes power.

Outboards are water cooled except for very-low-power units that air cool ribbed cylinders and water cool only the lower gear case. In all units an integral pump takes in water through immersed ports on the lower gear case that also houses bevel gears and clutch. Temperature control is by a thermostat in the engine block (see Thermostats).

Time was when outboard motors were restricted to "white" gasoline. Present-day manuacturers are agreed that their motors may be fueled with any automotive gasoline whose octane is at least 87 at the pump. The oil for the engine is a high-grade two-cycle lube, often the motor maker's own brand. (See Lubricating Oils.) The quality of the oil is one of the factors that decrees the ratio of gas and oil with which to fill the tank. The lower section of the gear housing is filled to the inspection hole with the gear case lubricant recommended by the owner's manual.

Outboard motors are high-speed machines. Maximum rated horsepower generally is obtained around 5,000 rpm. At speeds as high as this, perfect balance of all rotating parts is extremely important. Even a slight imbalance causes destructive vibration.

The outboard motor is capable of more effective steering of the boat than a rudder and fixed propeller. The reason is that the outboard thrust is aimed directly to the steering angle, while the thrust of the fixed prop is aimed by the rudder. The consequent two reactive forces are not equal.

A recent new feature for outboard motors is the use of counter-rotating propellers. The normal shaft carrying a single prop is replaced by two concentric shafts, each with a propeller. The props are directly behind each other and turn in opposite directions.

Present engine designs load the fuel mixture into the combustion chamber in either of two patterns: either "cross charge" or "loop charge." These names are self-explanatory. Each pattern has its staunch adherents who think it best.

Maintenance Maintenance of an outboard motor in running condition consists mostly of lubrication and of lube checks. A quick, clean manner of achieving the chosen ratio of oil and gasoline adds to the pleasure of running the boat. A squirt can is handy for lubricating all points where metal turns or slides upon metal. (See Lubricating Oils.)

The propeller should be checked for nicks and damage that can unbalance it; this is done best after removal of fouling and cleaning right down to shining metal (see Propellers). Cooling-water intake ports should be cleared. It is recommended that spark plugs be taken out at sensible intervals and checked for their condition (see Spark Plugs).

The fuel filter directly before the carburetor can become the source of annoying trouble if neglected. Whether or not it is to be replaced depends upon its type; some filters can be cleaned, others cannot. Observation and inspection should spot which is which. Clean with the correct solvent, and blow dry before reconnecting. (See Filters.)

What might be termed "pre-maintenance" is the routine prescribed by each manufacturer for the correct breaking-in of its outboard motor. The step-by-step routine is given in the appropriate owner's manual.

A general summary of the process reveals that for the first 15 minutes, the engine should not exceed its slowest cruising speed. The speed is to be increased to half-throttle for the next 45 minutes, and during this period short bursts of acceleration to full throttle are desirable. The following hour may be run at three-quarter throttle, again with short bursts. Unrestricted operation of the outboard motor is not deemed wise until this careful pattern has been followed for about a total of five hours.

There is one habit that every boatman in a powerboat should become addicted to: intermittent checking to make certain that cooling water is regularly flowing overboard. A quick glance over the stern to observe the water is all that is necessary. (Absence of the water is a serious omen and should trigger a shutdown.)

Troubleshooting Outboard troubleshooting logic: This a combination of an engine and a gearbox (transmission) and may present two separate problems. Solutions require a little savvy in both departments.

Shift in neutral, but starter rope will not pull out: Interlock pawl stuck (see Rope Starters).

Excessive smoke: Wrong gas/oil ratio. Wrong oil. Malfunction of the VRO (see Variable-Ratio Oiling). Carburetor float too high (see Carburetors).

Engine runs, but unit will not shift into forward or reverse: Check shift cable and rods. Corrosion. Clutch dog stuck on shaft (see Transmissions).

The breaker point condition and gap may be checked after removing the engine cover and the rope starter and flywheel. (Most late-model outboards are breakerless.)

Repair There is little the average boatman can do in the matter of repairs to an outboard motor. Lack of experience and skill is amplified by the lack of special tools. The growing use of metric screws and nuts becomes an added hurdle. Moreover, professional outboard-repair shops have test tanks in which they can make running adjustments and checks that duplicate conditions underway.

Paints

For the lovingly comforted wooden boat, relatively few of which are found these days, a skin of paint renewed annually is both cosmetic and protective.

PAINTS

For wooden boat owners, painting has long been one of the basic fine arts of boatkeeping. Now that fiberglass is more prevalent as a hull material, painting concerns the boatman less and less. Perhaps the only form of boat painting that now is almost universal is the application of an antifouling coat to the hull bottom.

Despite this decrease in the amount of painting of topsides, and in apparent contrast to it, recent years have brought fantastic improvements in boat paint. The new formulations grip and stay on better. They defy the sun better. They no longer are simple mixes of pigment, vehicle, and solvent. Modern boat paints are complicated chemical combinations that comprise amazing resins previously unavailable.

A few chemical technical terms must be understood as a forerunner to becoming comfortable with modern paints. The simplest and most common is "emulsion." An emulsion is a mixture of two substances that normally do not mix—as oil and water. The mix is accomplished with the aid of an "emulsifier" that creates an inner phase and an outer phase, one within the other. That oil and water do not mix is a basic fact of Nature. An emulsifier overcomes this. It breaks the oil into microscopic drops (the inner phase), each surrounded by a wall of water (the outer phase) that prevents coalescing (oil in water emulsion). When the water is the outer phase of an oil/water emulsion, then the mixture is soluble in water. An example is paint whose solvent is water and whose brushes wash clean with water. Application of this paint to a surface breaks the emulsion, leaving the water to evaporate while the pigment/resin remains as a coating. The absence of a flammable solvent vapor makes this type of coating a choice for application in enclosed spaces.

Resins are the body of paint and carry the pigment. Natural resins are the sap of trees, while synthetic resins are the products of chemical manipulation. Modern paint manufacture depends upon the synthetic resins.

The following are the synthetic resins most in vogue today with commercial boat paint manufacturers: Alkyds, modified alkyds, acrylics, epoxies, polyesters, isocyanates, urethanes, and polyurethanes. A "ballpark" generalization assigns the widest use and lowest prices to the alkyds. The acrylics are the plastics that substitute for glass, so naturally they add sparkle and clarity of color to paints. The polyesters find use in colored gelcoats, while the epoxies are limited to specialized coverings. The polyurethanes have become the star performers among synthetic resins because of the improved paints they have made possible.

The continuing disappearance of wooden boats from the pleasure-boating scene has caused a concomitant reduction in the use of the cosmetic coating called "varnish." Nevertheless, the warm glow of an expertly varnished rail and house (the brightwork) is still the pride of many a wooden boat owner.

Varnish is an unpigmented combination of resin and solvent. It is transparent when applied and brings out the beauty in wood. Unlike paint (which is "worked out"), varnish is laid down in long, flowing strokes that give a hard glaze to the surface (see

PAINTS

Varnishes). The sun is the enemy of varnish, and many varnish formulations contain anti-solar, "UV-protection" ingredients. When the wood surface is unattractive, it may be improved by using a stain (pigment in a solvent) or a filler (pigment paste) prior to varnishing.

When a series of coating products is used in carrying out a complete paint job, it is wise to select all of them from the same manufacturer. This eliminates the possibility of one coat "picking up" a previous coat: A paint (resin) can "pick up" a previous coat of paint (resin) over which it is spread, through the combined action of solvency and chemical cross-linking. Furthermore, purchasing products from one manufacturer provides a source for help and a destination for complaints. Nor should the wealth of information on the can label be ignored.

The days when any paint could be brushed over any other paint are gone. The highly specialized paint chemistry of today requires careful reading of the paint can label—and even a call to the paint manufacturer when in doubt. Consider unfriendly paints to be like cats and dogs.

Paints may be selected on the basis of their surface finish. This may be either matte, semi-gloss, or gloss. Gloss is the easiest to keep clean, but it has the bad habit of accentuating blemishes in the surface. As for color, white is the always-acceptable boat color, and it flatters most boats. Most skippers fear dark-colored hulls because of rub-off with accidental contact.

An entire class of paints is devoted to the never-ending battle between the boatman and the plants and animals that want to stake out a home site on the ship's bottom. These paints are called antifouling coatings. They are heavily loaded with a poison, such as copper, that slowly disperses into the surrounding water. (Tributyltin as a poison has been outlawed.) The cost of these paints relates to the percentage of poisonous copper they contain; vinyl is a popular vehicle. The span of time over which an antifouling paint is effective depends upon many factors; most skippers repaint every year.

The diminishing number of wooden boats leaves fewer and fewer boats to be painted because the fiberglass vessels rarely need this drastic attention. For boats that do need painting, a few pointers follow.

Contrary to the thinking of the average inexperienced boatman, the hard part of the work of painting, and the greater consumer of time, lies in preparation of the surface. (One manufacturer found upon investigation that almost every complaint of improper finish could be traced to negligent preparation.) Slapping the brush around is actually the fun part. A good craftsman will devote three-quarters of every hour of painting time to the energetic use of sandpaper (see Sandpaper). The market offers so-called "no-sand" liquids; avoid them, because there is no substitute for sandpaper and elbow grease.

What type of first coat to apply to a wooden hull after the surface has been properly sanded depends on the nature of the wood. Some woods do not present a surface suitable for adhesion of paint directly. These woods must first be "primed" with a formulation called a primer that acts as an interface. Prim-

PAINTS

ers are available not only for wood but also for metal and fiberglass. Another pre-paint formulation is the "undercoat." This coating is purposely loaded with finely powdered mineral filler that sands away easily to aid in making a smooth surface for the subsequent paint.

It is not always necessary to "get down to the wood." If the previous paint has held well, a thorough sanding should provide an adequate base for the new paint. The simple trick is to follow the instructions on the can, on the assumption that the manufacturer is most knowledgeable of the product.

The sandings that precede the coat of actual paint should be done with dry paper. The starting numbers of the grits should be in the 90s, and the finishing numbers should be in the 200s. Subsequent sanding of the paint should be done with wet-and-dry paper and water. Several sheets of paper should be soaking themselves clean while one sheet is being used. Sandpaper has become expensive, and this system increases its life greatly.

When it comes to application of paint, the question arises of brush versus roller. On a wooden vessel, especially for the early coats, the brush is better. With fiberglass and metal boats, a good roller twirler can equal brush quality and save time. It is a valid assumption that most skippers handle a wheel better than a paintbrush, and they should consider professional assistance—certainly with a hull that has been coated with any of the urethane or isocyanate paints.

There comes a time when paint must be removed. Three methods are at hand: sanding, burning, and chemical removal. There is nothing wrong with sanding except the time, effort, and mountains of sandpaper it consumes. Burning is murderous to wood, a no-no for fiberglass, and it can harm metal. Chemical removal with a paint remover is the acceptable practice and entails the least amount of work.

Several good paint removers are available on the market, and, if possible, the choice should be a nonflammable one that is not runny. To get the most mileage out of a remover, it should be brushed on and left until the paint blisters and lifts. A putty knife is the handiest tool for removing lifted paint. Working in the shade is preferable, because the sun dries up the remover and tends to paste the loosened paint right back onto the surface. Safety-minded workers use gloves and goggles. Paint removers, like all paint products, are deleterious to health, and the precautions found on most paint can labels should be followed; common sense is the guide. Be sure to dispose of the toxic chemical waste properly.

The residue of paint removers can prevent good adhesion of subsequent paint and must be cleaned away thoroughly. Cleanup may be as simple as a water washdown, or it may even require chemical means; the answer direct from the horse's mouth is on the can.

Shellac and lacquer coatings are not usually found on a boat, but a word about them may come in handy. Both shellac and lacquer are simple solutions of a resin in a solvent. For shellac, the solvent is alcohol; for lacquer it is lacquer thinner, an acetone-like liquid. Both coatings may be reliquified and washed away by application of their solvents. (The adhesiveness and water resistance of shellac can make it serve as a bedding compound for flat surfaces in an emergency.)

Antifouling paint is a poison and should be treated as such during application and especially if it is being sanded, following the precautions stated on the can or by the manufacturer. Although the copper is in a finely divided state, it is believed, nevertheless, to act like a homogeneous metal and to set up electrolysis (see Electrolysis). This requires countermeasures when the copper antifouling is painted on a metal hull. The usual action is to underlay a coat of electrically insulating barrier paint.

A comparison reading of manufacturers' paint coverage figures seems to emphasize the numbers 300 and 500. These designate the square feet of surface that may be covered per gallon. The 300 refers to primers, while the 500 describes finish coats. Most paints will fall between those two areas. (These are "ballpark" figures, but should prove of some help.)

An engine cleaned with one of the commercial "gooks" and then washed down with warm, soapy water and painted will look beautifully yachty. Engine manufacturers can supply pressurized spray cans of their trademark colors.

Maintenance Little in the form of maintenance need be done for painted surfaces other than to keep them clean. A thorough freshwater hosing after each boat trip to remove salt and grime fulfills the requirement. Some paints are formulated to chalk and renew their surface, but these are generally house paints and out of place on a boat.

Personal Flotation Devices

The official Coast Guard designation is "personal flotation devices." To the average boatman, they are "life jackets" or "life savers." By whatever name, both the law and common sense mandate that these "PFDs" be aboard in legally specified quantity and style.

The Coast Guard divides personal flotation devices into five types. The required effective buoyancy for each type also is listed. This matter of buoyancy may need explanation: A person who has fallen into the water generally does not automatically float, because his natural buoyancy is not equal to his weight. As an example, a 170-pounder may have a buoyancy of only 160 pounds, and he will sink unless a PFD supplies the missing 10 pounds or more. Thus, the Coast Guard sets the required buoyancy for each type of PFD. Type I must have a buoyancy of 20 pounds, Type II of 15½ pounds, Type III of 15½ pounds, Type IV of 16½ pounds, and Type V of unspecified amount.

PFD Type I is the top of the line, with the greatest buoyancy, and, in addition, it has the ability to turn its wearer's face up out of the water. The design of Type II makes it more comfortable to wear and yet retains the major features of Type I. In both Type I and Type II PFDs, it is expected that

PERSONAL FLOTATION DEVICES

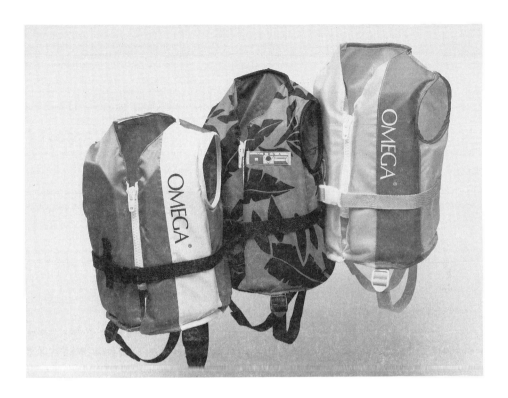

PERSONAL FLOTATION DEVICES—These are PFDs for children. (A child's PFD must provide a minimum buoyancy of 7 pounds.) Most young children think wearing a PFD is fun. *(Courtesy Omega)*

turning the face out of the water will take place even if the wearer is unconscious.

The Type III PFD will keep its wearer vertical in the water, but he is expected to consciously maintain that position. The Type IV PFD is throwable and is expected to be grabbed and hung onto and not necessarily worn. Type V is a catch-all for a variety of life-preserving devices.

The flotation material in PFDs may be kapok, or fibrous glass, or specified plastic foams; the regulations specify how loose material must be encased, for instance, in sealed bags. PFDs carry the manufacturer's name and address, Coast Guard approval number, and details of inspection. The color must be international orange. Jackets, vests, and other forms must meet the applicable type requirements. Note that previous models of PFDs, which do not contain their flotation material in sealed plastic bags, are no longer legal.

PFDs are available in a size for adults and a size for children, and they are marked accordingly and ummistakably. (A popular mail-order marine catalog lists a PFD for a dog that may be had in several sizes.)

It is a good rule for children to re-

PLOTTING

main in their PFDs for as long as they are aboard. The law requires that each vessel carry at least one PFD for each person carried. Boats more than 26 feet long must add one throwable Type IV. PFDs should be stored *out* of their plastic shipping bags and in a location accessible in the direst emergency.

Repair Personal flotation devices are not repairable. Any damage or deterioration to a PFD immediately cancels its legality and prohibits its further use.

Plotting

Plotting is the art of representing the actual or the desired track of a vessel on a chart by means of vectors, lines of specified length and direction. A representative problem solved by plotting

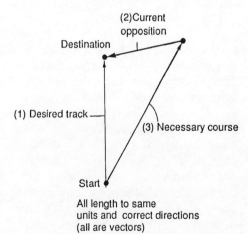

All length to same units and correct directions (all are vectors)

PLOTTING—Plotting is an easily acquired skill and a handy one for the skipper to possess. (See text; also Vectors.)

entails finding the course to steer when an off-setting current affects the progress of the boat (see Vectors).

The current and boat speed and heading may be interacting in one of three ways: (1) The current is in line with the boat track and running in the same direction. (Add current speed to boat speed.) (2) The current is in line with the boat track but running in the opposite direction. (Subtract current speed from boat speed.) (3) The current is at any other angle with boat track. (A graphic vectorial solution gives the answer.)

The illustration details how one skipper used vectors to arrive at the best course to steer. The start and the destination are directly opposite on the north and south banks of a wide river. The current is at an angle that prevents a straight-across steering.

Line 1 is drawn from start to finish and is divided into as many parts as equals boat speed. Line 2 is laid down to exact current direction and correct length in the same speed units. Line 3 closes the vector triangle and shows the course to steer. This line also shows SOG (speed over the ground) and SOA (speed of advance) with slight additional drawing.

Polarity (Electric)

Often the need arises to determine whether an available circuit is alternating current (AC) or direct current (DC)—and, if the latter, what its polarity is. The answer may be found quickly with the aid of a glass of water.

PREAMPLIFIERS

PREAMPLIFIERS—Preamplifiers may be located at the head end of receivers or directly at the antenna for greatest effectiveness. The preamp in the circuit shown is at the antenna for greatest effectiveness in overcoming local electrical noises. Note the separate ground.

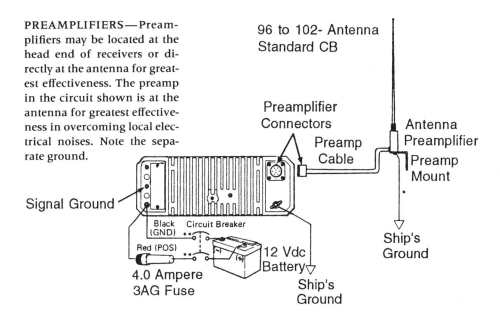

Immerse the two bared wires of the doubtful circuit, keeping them about ½ or more inch apart. An alternating current will cause both wires to give off bubbles. With direct current, only the negative wire will make bubbles.

If the voltage is very low and the bubbling consequently faint, the indications will be improved by a dash of salt in the water.

Careful! Touching the wires together will cause a short circuit!

Preamplifiers

A radio preamplifier is exactly what its name implies: an amplifier located at the input to strengthen a received signal before it is fed to the main circuit. Thus strengthened, the signal can more effectively overcome local noise and maintain the clarity of its information.

Preamplifiers are located at the input of receiver circuits. Often they are a separate cabinet at the antenna; in this position they help overcome noises picked up inadvertently by the lead-in wire.

Preamplifiers are staffed with transistors especially designed to produce negligible internal noise during operation (see Transistors). Noise (electrical noise) is the limiting factor in determining the weakest signal that may be handled successfully.

Preamplifiers may also contain sharp tuning circuits that assist in narrowing reception down to a desired frequency (see VHF-FM Radios). For some services, preamplifiers may be variably tuned.

Modern miniature transistors enable many preamplifiers to be condensed to a small section of circuit board.

Propellers

A propeller does not "push against the water," as is commonly believed. A propeller is a reactive device and follows Nature's law, "Every action has an equal and opposite reaction." Forcing a mass of water rearward is the propeller's action. The consequent forward thrust of the boat is the reaction.

The shape of a propeller and its blades is familiar. Although there may be slight dissimilarities to achieve an individual designer's goals, all propellers are reasonably alike but may differ in the number of blades balanced around a central hub. The convex/concave shape of the blade is most efficient in imparting mainly axial velocity to the water with a minimum of useless spiral velocity.

The least number of blades on a propeller is two; the most is five (rarely, six). The curvature of the blade face, the pitch, is cut by special machines, and the surface is polished to reduce the friction of the water passing over it. The two-blade propeller is a favorite for sailboats because it may be lined up behind the keel, out of the way when sailing without power; the reduction of drag is significant. The two-blade propeller is also available with blades that fold out of the way.

Unfortunately, a propeller also generates undesirable side thrust that can affect steering, especially when backing with a single-screw. The cause lies with the angle of the propeller shaft, and the resultant tilt from the vertical of the propeller. Although the blades are identical, the blade going down acts as though it were different in pitch from the blade coming up. Technically, it is a dissimilarity in the angle of attack, and this brings side thrust.

Propellers are manufactured from plastic, steel, aluminum, and bronze. The popular choice seems to be bronze. Propellers are called "right-hand" or "left-hand." The right-hand propeller turns clockwise when viewed from astern of the boat, the left-hand coun-

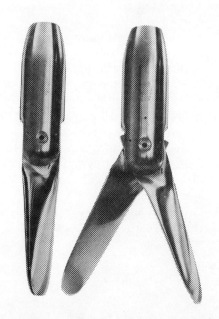

PROPELLERS—The propeller transforms engine power into thrust. The folding model relieves sailboats of drag when running on sail alone. Centrifugal force aligns the folded blades into working position. *(Courtesy Michigan Wheel)*

PROPELLERS

terclockwise. On a twin-screw boat, the preference is a left-hand prop to port and a right-hand prop to starboard. (The tops of the propellers are turning away from each other.)

A condition may develop in which the surfaces of the propeller lose their "hold" on the water, even though the propeller is still submerged. This is equivalent to spinning the prop in a vacuum, divorced from its load, and causing the engine to overspeed, often dangerously. This unwanted condition is known as "cavitation." Miniature "sonic booms" also take place and pockmark the surfaces of the propeller (see Cavitation).

Propeller specifications are hub diameter, overall diameter, pitch, left or right, number of blades, and material. Some propeller hubs are designed to pass engine exhaust. Pitch is the theoretical distance the prop would advance in one revolution.

The original specifications for the propeller of a hull are the designer's job and entail intricate calculations. However, after the pencil pushing is completed, a correct solution may still depend upon trial and error.

Technically speaking, the right propeller will load the engine to its listed maximum speed. Overspeeding at load may require an increase in pitch or in diameter; inability to reach the engine's listed speed takes the opposite treatment. The reduction gear also enters the problem.

Variable-pitch propellers give the skipper great latitude in melding the requirements of engine, propeller, and hull and thus receive full benefit from every gallon of fuel. In the variable-pitch construction, a control rod reaches the prop hub through a hollow shaft and swings the blade's surfaces from the forward position through neutral to reverse. (A reverse gear is not needed.)

Maintenance The efficiency of a propeller depends on strict observance of the polished working surfaces. Propellers should be examined at every opportunity for the presence of pock marks, indicative of cavitation (see Cavitation). On larger boats it may be financially worthwhile to hire a diver to go down and do a prop-cleaning job.

Troubleshooting Keep a sharp lookout to prevent "fouling" the propeller (the tangling of a line, net, or other object around it). It is quite possible for a speeding propeller to break a shaft if it becomes suddenly stopped by an enwinding line. This can be prevented by installation of a device called a rope cutter (see Rope Cutter).

The almost universal cause of damage to a prop is grounding of the boat. This is especially true when there is no protecting skeg. The usual damage to the prop consists of torn blade edges and bent blades. A damaged propeller is an unbalanced wheel, and running it could cause dangerous vibrations, so don't delay in getting it repaired.

Repair Luckily, propeller repairers have become expert in returning stricken props to good health. Most marinas have reciprocal arrangements with propeller shops in their area. In most cases this establishes an exchange policy for the skipper. The damaged prop, plus a fee, can be exchanged for a rebuilt propeller without the necessity of waiting for the repair. The prop shop checks the replacement for exact duplication of specifications.

Radar Reflectors

Small boats traveling in or near commercial shipping lanes are in danger of being run down unless they can announce their presence to the behemoths by appearing on their radar screens. Luckily, it is easy to accomplish this without having any equipment on the small boat other than a radar reflector. Reflectors are passive devices requiring no power.

Radar waves are short and reflect from surfaces as light waves would. As with light, some surfaces are more reflective than others, and radar reflectors are designed to have greater reflective ability than wooden and fiberglass hulls.

The reflector is hoisted high in the rigging. Hopefully, at least one of the reflective surfaces is always at an angle that will bounce back some of the powerful radar energy striking it. These bounces become pips on the big ship's wheelhouse screens. (Whether or not the watch takes note is in the hands of the gods.)

Radar reflectors are manufactured of plastic and metal laminates that are good reflectors. The mechanical design is often collapsible for storage. They are reasonably resistant to wind and rain and should be flown as high as possible.

Radars

A radar installation uses bursts of extremely short radio waves to achieve RAdio Detection And Ranging. The radio waves are reflected back by their targets to produce "pips" on the radar screen. The location of the pip on the screen imparts the desired distance and azimuth information. (Azimuth is the horizontal angle between a fixed point and an observed object.)

The radar system comprises two parts: the antenna unit and the display unit, connected by multi-wire, shielded cable. The antenna rotates continuously while the system is in use. The display unit in many small radars has replaced the familiar television-type tube with a liquid crystal screen that is simpler, more compact, and has thousands of pixels per square inch for high-resolution pictures. The instantaneous direction in which the antenna points and the azimuth indication on the screen are maintained in absolute agreement.

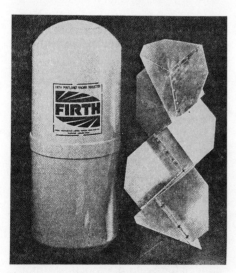

RADAR REFLECTORS—A radar reflector. In this design, the actual reflector unit (right) fits inside the protective case (left).

RADARS

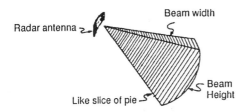

RADARS—The theoretical shape of the beam projected by the radar antenna. The beam is narrow in its horizontal dimension to ensure separation of targets, and wide vertically to compensate for ship's roll.

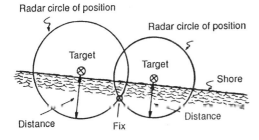

RADAR—Two radar measurements are easily plotted as a fix.

The sequence of events that constitutes a radar cycle starts with the generation of the extremely high-frequency radio waves in the antenna unit. The antenna is connected to the transmitter, and a short burst of energy is directed at the target. The antenna is immediately connected to the receiver to catch the radio echo. (The switching back and forth of the antenna is done electronically.) The echo pulse is directed at the screen and forms a pip. Reference to the scale and to the angle gives the distance and the azimuth of the target.

The number of times per second that this cycle takes place is the "pulse repetition rate" (PRR) of the radar. Since the PRR must allow time for the transmission and for the echo, it is slowed for long-distance ranging, which requires greater energy bursts and longer travel time. (The description "slowed" is purely relative, because the time periods involved are only fractions of one-millionth of one second.) The duration of each pulse within the pulse train determines how much energy hits the target and therefore how much is available for the echo. Typically, the PRR lies between 1,000 and 2,000.

The shape of the beam emitted by the antenna may be envisioned as a slice of pie standing on edge with its point at the antenna. The width of the beam in a horizontal directionn is approximately 2 degrees; it is kept narrow so as to separate the targets. The width of the pie in a vertical direction is approximately 30 degrees; this is to maintain coverage of the target while the ship rolls.

The true radar pips that designate targets on the screen are often inundated and confused by pips called "clutter." Weather clutter is caused by echoes from rain and snow, and a "fast time constant" (FTC) is provided to control it. Sea clutter, echoes from waves, is controlled by a "short time constant" (STC). (If not carefully set, these two controls can wipe out the pips from true targets.)

Manufacturers rate their radars with two specifications that often confuse the skipper into considering his radar to be more powerful than it actually is: effective range, and total power. The range is given in miles, the power in kilowatts; both are always optimistic.

Take a unit advertised as a "35-mile

RADAR REFLECTORS

radar." Even assuming it has the requisite power, it cannot function at this range unless it is mounted high enough above the waterline to have a 35-mile line of sight.

This same radar probably would be labeled as having "3.5 kilowatts" of "peak effective power" (PEP). Clearly, 3,500 watts cannot be drawn continuously from the storage battery. Further checking establishes that the real power of the unit is 85 watts and requires only 7 amperes from the battery. The PEP rating is based on a full-power beam for only the period of less than one-millionth of one second.

Antenna rotation is approximately 20 revolutions per minute, and the beam on the screen is, of course, in synchronism (see Antennas). Early radars had parabolic reflectors serving as their antennas, with great similarity to a searchlight except for the substitution of invisible waves for waves of light. Modern radar antennas are slotted wave guides, simpler and more efficient. For sailboats, the rotating portion of the antenna is in a plastic housing that prevents snagging on the rigging. (Plastic is transparent to radio.)

Constant practice is the key to becoming sufficiently familiar with the radar to enable its use in foulweather navigation. The practicing is done in clear daylight when the pip on the screen and the equivalent target may be seen and compared simultaneously. It becomes largely a matter of memory, because there is little relationship between the pip and whatever the radar beam echoed from. The "picture" on the screen may be considered a shadowgraph.

Old-time radars had screens large enough and accessible enough to permit course plotting directly on the glass with a grease pencil. Today's plotting had best be done on printed sheets called "maneuvering boards." These are supplied in pads of 50 sheets and bear the identification "2665-10,HO." Each sheet is imprinted with angular scales and distance scales that make it easy to mark down the radar information and then work to a conclusion of the navigational problem. (See Maneuvering Boards.)

Repair Any repair or adjustment of the radar unit most likely will involve work on the oscillator/transmitter and, by law, this must be done by a properly licensed radar technician. A quick check to verify that the unit is functioning may be made, legally, with a small fluorescent tube such as is found in desk lamps. The tube should glow when held directly in front of the operating antenna.

Ranges

A range provides an optical centerline for a channel. With proper observation and steering, a helmsman can run the center of the channel fairway simply by holding the two range markers like the front and rear sights of a gun.

The value of a range is illustrated dramatically by one area where a wide river crosses the Intracoastal Waterway (ICW) at right angles. A wide expanse of unmarked water results, but a range becomes visible. Holding the

RANGES

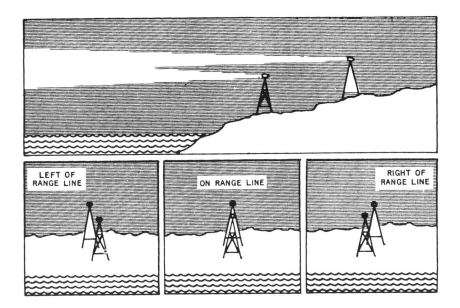

RANGES—A helmsman's eye view of a range in use is shown. *(Courtesy U.S. Coast Guard)* Range lights may be white, red, or green, and display various characteristics to differentiate them from surrounding lights.

range on "zero" makes crossing the river easy and leads directly to the continuation of the ICW markers. Ranges also find some use by marinas and boatyards to direct traffic incoming from the main stream without the need for markers.

Ranges consist of long, narrow, rectangular panels, vertically striped and vertically placed on raised platforms. The front range is lower than the rear, and the size is determined by the distance over which they must be viewed. The front range is geographically located on the chart; the rear range is located in degrees and distance from the front range. The true bearing of the range centerline may also be shown.

Ranges can, of course, be created by anyone with a good chart showing towers, tanks, spires, etc.

Some of the more important ranges are lighted to provide extended usage. Either red, green, or white lights may be used. (The normal background lighting of built-up shore areas may make range lights a bit difficult to distinguish and flashing patterns may be used.)

The range panels give the helmsman more than merely centerline information. By observing which range first comes into view, he can tell whether the boat is to the right or to the left of the centerline. For both optical and local reasons, a range may be fully usable for only a portion of its full length, and this distance will be marked by buoys.

When fully on the range, the rear range stripes will become continuous with the front range stripes.

REFRIGERATION

Refrigeration

Mechanical refrigeration has become a standard comfort on all pleasure boats that have a galley. Mates no longer tolerate the mess and bother of bringing ice aboard. Small, compact, electric refrigerators designed for marine service are widely available at reasonable cost. Conversion units, intended for do-it-yourself installation, modernize the old icebox and eliminate the need for ice.

Consider mechanical refrigeration equipment as a machine for extracting heat from food, thereby cooling it, and then dissipating this heat into the galley. (In the icebox, the heat from food went into the drip water from the melting ice.) All of this refrigerating gear has the capability of producing the ice cubes so necessary for the happy cruising of many skippers.

The complete refrigeration system consists of a motor-driven compressor, a condenser, an evaporator, a capillary tube, and various filters and driers. These units are all connected in series, one after the other. The system is charged with a fluorocarbon chemical called Freon. The evaporator is located in the freezer compartment; the remaining units are placed where convenient and nearby. (Freon is chosen because of the efficient manner in which it can be vaporized and condensed in the refrigeration cycle.) The megayachts all have separate freezers, like large households.

Both the small refrigerators and the conversion units are built to run on either the 12-volt boat battery or the 120-volt power line. Two separate, noninterchangeable power cords protect against mistaken plugging into the wrong source of electricity. The current drain when running on the battery is approximately 5 amperes; off the power line, the drain is about 60 watts.

The installation of conversion units is not difficult and requires no more technical knowledge than is found in the owner's manual. The units are charged with Freon at the factory. Without this precharge, a long and thorough vacuum pumpdown would be necessary to remove all air. Air inside the closed piping system is the enemy of efficient refrigeration.

Understanding the operation of the system helps greatly in getting the best service from it. The repetitious action starts at the compressor that puts the Freon under pressure and sends it to the condenser. The condenser removes the heat of compression and allows the Freon to return to liquid form. The liquid goes on to the evaporator via the capillary tube that restricts the flow to a designed amount. The evaporator is maintained at low pressure by the suction of the compressor, causing the liquid Freon to flash to a gas. The gas is drawn into the compressor, and the cycle is repeated as long as refrigeration is called for by the fridge thermostat.

That change of state from liquid to gas and back again is the secret of mechanical refrigeration. The vaporization from liquid to gas cannot take place without the addition of heat—and this is the heat taken from the food. During the change from gas to liquid, heat is given off, and this is the heat the condenser dissipates to the ambient air. This must be considered

ROPE CUTTER

when installing the equipment: The condenser must have access to plenty of air.

The quality and the amount of the insulation are equally important for the efficiency of the mechanical equipment. (This caution of necessity applies only to conversion installations, because the manufactured refrigerators are beyond change by the buyer.) Conversion installation instructions provide much detailed how-to that should be followed in the purchase and placement of insulation. A primary requisite is insulation that does not absorb moisture.

Installation As already noted, refrigeration must be installed in a manner that will assure plenty of air circulation for the condenser. Discharge must also be provided for the condensate water that collects in the food compartment. (In standard refrigerators this is boiled off by a condenser coil under the cabinet.)

Generally, the drip water lands in the bilge. This is not good practice. In wooden hulls, this leads to rot. In fiberglass hulls, it may become a source of bad odor. A weep hole for overboard discharge is an excellent idea, if possible.

Troubleshooting A correctly functioning refrigerator should be making ice cubes—and monitoring this is one form of troubleshooting. Occasional reference to a refrigeration thermometer in the food compartment is recommended; the reading should be around 42 degrees Fahrenheit.

Repair The servicing of refrigerators is not complicated and could be within the ken of handy skippers, except for the special tools and gauges required. Thus, most breakdowns will mean a call for a technician.

One exception could be poor refrigeration because of a tiny leak of Freon. Adding Freon carefully at what is called the "suction side valve" (on the compressor intake side) could restore normal operation for a period of time. The Freon is added slowly and carefully while the unit is running. Frost on the suction line signals Freon overdose. Supply stores sell small cans of Freon plus the needed tubing and adapter valve. The Freon must be identical with that in the unit. The type of Freon may be stated on the unit's nameplate.

Rope Cutter

A chance encounter with a length of rogue rope winding itself around (fouling) the propeller usually means an immediate haulout or the services of an experienced diver. Lucky is the skipper in this predicament who does not also find a broken shaft. The forces involved in this sudden stoppage are so great that damage may reach all the way into the engine.

A unique device known as a rope cutter claims to avoid all rogue rope damage by immediately cutting away the offending rope.

Installation The rope cutter is installed at the propeller. A sharp, vee-shaped blade attaches to the prop bearing. A mating blade, attached to the propeller, flashes by and acts like a shear.

ROPE STARTERS

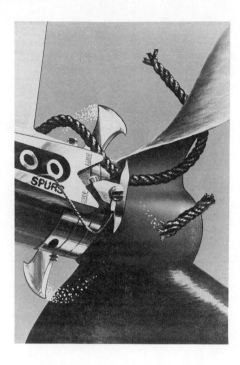

ROPE CUTTER—This device is insurance against the damage that may be caused by a rogue rope picked up by the propeller and wound around the shaft. A broken shaft in such a situation is not unusual. *(Courtesy Spurs Marine)*

Rope Starters

For many years, yanking on a rope was the only way to start an outboard motor. Then, as increasing horsepowers raised the required yank beyond average strength, the electric starter became an integral part of the big outboard. Still today, the lower horsepowers retain the rope.

The heart of the rope starter is a powerful coil spring. This spring retracts the rope when it reaches the end of its travel and rewinds it ready for the next pull. The rope starter and the engine are in rotational contact only during the actual pull; when the engine fires, it over-runs the starter and the two become entirely disconnected rotationally.

The rope starter incorporates an important safety feature: A pawl locks the starter and prevents the engine from starting unless the gear shift is in neutral. This interlocking is accomplished by a cable connection to the shift mechanism.

When the rope is pulled, a pawl extends from the rope pulley and jams against the cup attached to the engine flywheel. Thus, the two turn together and the engine starts. The engine speed retracts the pawl and allows the rope pulley to rewind when the rope is released. If the engine fails to fire, additional pulls on the rope may be made in quick succession as long as the gear shift is not moved from neutral.

Maintenance In all probability, the most maintenance the rope starter will need over a lifetime is judicious lubrication and a replacement of the rope. The extendable pawl must swing easily and must move freely on its pin. The exact length of rope needed is noted in the owner's manual.

Troubleshooting Troubleshooting logic: Pulling the rope should lock the starter and the engine together; releasing the rope should separate them.
Rope pulled, engine does not turn: Stuck pawl in rope pulley.
Rope pulled, engine starts, rope does not rewind: Broken spring. Unhooked spring.
Starter not locked out in forward and reverse: Safety pawl not working. Check cable to shift. Pawl corroded (dangerous condition).

Repair To replace the rope, first remove the engine cover and the screws holding the starter to the engine. Release the spring, but do not remove it, and remove the rope pulley. Remove the rope handle. *Beware of injury from coiled spring.* When reassembling, make sure that the spring hook is around the drive pin.

Rudder Indicators

A helmsman taking over the wheel without knowing the position of the rudder may find himself in a dangerous situation when he applies power to get underway. He does not know what the immediate reaction of the boat will be. A rudder position indicator provides insurance against such a scenario.

The rudder indicator monitors rudder angle constantly and displays its findings on a small meter on the console. A three-terminal variable resistor (a potentiometer) is the sensor on the rudderpost. The indicator is actually a center-zero voltmeter. These two devices, plus a few resistors, attaching brackets, and connecting wire, make up the system. The wiring diagram is shown in the illustration. It takes two people to check a rudder indicator, one at the instrument and the other at the rudder, checking indicated against actual position.

The circuit of the rudder indicator is technically known as a "bridge" circuit. It works on the principle of balance and unbalance in either a positive or a negative direction. With the rudder centered amidships, the circuit is in balance; no current flows, and the meter remains at center zero. With the rudder off center, there is unbalance, and either positive or negative current flows through the meter, with consequent meter-needle swing in the rudder direction.

The meter may be calibrated in degrees of rudder swing, but this generally is superfluous for a small boat, although valuable information for big ships.

The rudder indicator system works off the 12-volt boat battery. The electrical resistance of the rudder indicator is high, and this keeps the current drawn down to a negligible value.

Maintenance The connecting links between potentiometer and rudderpost are adjustable and provide the means of making rudder arc agree with the meter calibration.

Rudders

As noted elsewhere in the text, "A boat going forward steers like an automobile going backward." The stern must be moved to the right in order to turn the bow to the left (see Bow Thrusters). The movements of the stern are initiated by the action of the rudder.

The rudder is a plane surface, normally at the end of the keel, mounted to swing on a vertical rudderpost. The amount of swing, from left to right, is under the control of the steering system and its tiller or wheel. The area of the plane surface of the rudder is closely calculated to the size and characteristics of the hull.

RULES OF THE ROAD

The rudder is a passive element; it has no power of its own. The turning force it exerts on the hull is reactive, the result of relative movement of the water and the rudder. In other words, the rudder must be moving against the water, or the water must be moving against the rudder. In either case, considerable turning force may be required. The source of the force may be human effort, with the added mechanical advantage of tiller or steering wheel; electro-mechanical or hydraulic (autopilots); or the wind (self-steerers).

The effectiveness of rudders, namely degree of ship turn per degree of rudder turn, is affected by wind, speed, and current. A skilled helmsman compensates for this subconsciously. Autopilots have a control to counteract sea conditions.

On multi-propeller boats, it is customary to place a rudder abaft each prop. Rudders generally are not called upon to serve in close docking procedures with multi-prop boats. "Steering" is done with variations of engine speed and direction.

Much experimenting has been done with rudder shape, but no absolute rule seems to have been reached. A check of production boats finds a variety of shapes. It is customary to have skeg support the lower corner of the rudder, although unsupported spade designs also are seen.

Rudder action on a powerboat differs from the action of the rudder on a sailboat without power. The powerboat rudder may have energy imparted to it by the propeller even when the vessel has no way on ("way on" is the boatman's term for moving forward or backward), and this may be used to "kick the stern around." The powerless sailboat has a dead rudder until the boat moves either forward or backward. In both cases, action results only after the rudder is turned into the stream of water. A rudder exerts directive effort only when water is moving against it.

Hydraulic and electric-motor devices (autopilots) are available to take over the work of moving the rudder back and forth (see Autopilots). Interesting also are the attempts to make the rudder a "servo" system with the addition of rudder tabs. (The automobile brake is an illustration of the servo principle: A small amount of the energy represented by the moving car is drained off and made to apply the brakes.) In the servo rudder, the energy the trim tab receives from the moving stream is used to turn the rudder; the steering system controls only the servo rudder or trim tab (see Trim Tabs).

Another scheme presents the balanced rudder. The vertical pivot is not at the rudder's forward edge, but is moved a short distance back. A portion of the water stream is thereby made to balance the main force.

Maintenance Wooden rudders of propeller-driven boats are subject to erosion by the high-velocity water streams or "prop wash." Rudder stuffing boxes need inspection for leaks (see Stuffing Boxes).

Rules of the Road

This is a digest of that portion of the Rules of the Road most likely to be in greatest use by skippers in popular boating areas.

Covered here are the following situations: head-on, passing, crossing, overtaking. The whistle signals indicated are to be given only when the boats are in actual sight of each other. In most situations, sailboats have the right of way over powerboats. Sailboats do not give whistle signals. Each rule determines which of the two boats concerned is the "stand-on" boat and which is the "give-way" boat.

Two boats are head-on when each skipper sees the other boat's red and green lights at night and, by day, when the two lubber lines would merge if extended. The skippers' choice is whether to pass port to port or starboard to starboard. The port choice requires one blast and a shift of course to the right. The starboard choice requires two blasts and a shift of course to the left. Either skipper may originate the choice, with the other agreeing by sounding an identical blast. (If the second skipper considers the move unsafe, he may sound the danger signal of five or more short blasts.)

When the course of one boat will cross the course of another (see Maneuvering Boards) and the danger of collision exists, the boat on the right has the right of way and becomes the stand-on boat. The stand-on boat continues on its course, and the give-way boat is required to stay out of the way.

The skipper of a boat wishing to overtake another blows one blast if he wishes to pass on the forward boat's starboard side, or two blasts if the pass is to be on the forward boat's port side. The forward boat replies with an identical signal to signify agreement. If, in the opinion of the forward boat, the move would be unsafe, the danger signal stops the overtaking.

The Rules of the Road have the purpose of preventing collisions at sea. They are not an invitation to whistle blowing.

(The foregoing just skims the rules. Every skipper should have at hand Coast Guard publication No. M-16672;2A which explains the rules clearly.)

Rust

Rust is expected on iron and steel fittings, but it comes as a surprise to find rust on stainless steel. The indictment is eased somewhat, and the reputation of stainless is maintained, by calling the smoothly adhering rust a "stain." This stain/rust may be removed by chemical application and by polishing. The procedure is basically the same for plain iron and steel, and for stainless, but it takes less work to clear stainless.

The overriding caution is *never* to polish with steel wool. The fact is, steel wool should *never* even be found on a boat. The tiny, almost invisible "splinters" that break away from steel wool in use, lodge in the deck and rust and defy removal.

Bronze wool is an acceptable substitute; even better is the use of the cutting compound employed in automobile shops. This is a compound of grease and emery powder, easily cleaned off with gasoline. It is "worked" with a tough rag, and the finer grades leave a dull, smooth surface, easily buffed to a shine with wax.

SAILS

Chemical removal of rust invariably calls on phosphoric acid diluted to about 5 percent. For convenience in use, the acid is made into a paste with a binder like cornstarch. Never wash up with water containing household bleach; the chlorine will mark the stainless.

Rust is an iron oxide, formed by the chemical combination of the iron with oxygen from the air, a sort of ultra-slow combustion.

Wherever practical, rust may be prevented by shutting off the oxygen with a surface sealant such as clear lacquer. This is applied instead of the wax polish after stain removal. The lacquer is available in self-spray cans.

Sails

As with rope, so also with sails: Synthetics have taken over, and sails of the natural fibers, such as cotton and flax, are rarely seen. Present-day sails are cut from Dacron. (Nylon, as sail material, is merely a runner-up.)

Dacron's preeminence as sail material is well earned. Contrary to cotton, Dacron absorbs negligible amounts of water. It does not rot if stowed wet. It is tougher and stronger. It stretches less than nylon and much less than cotton.

Relatively stretchless Dacron eliminates the constant adjustments of outhaul and halyard that become necessary with cotton sails when the weather changes. The greater strength of Dacron sails allows them to stay up in heavier weather.

Since Dacron is a harder material, Dacron sails are more subject to chafing against spars, shrouds, and stays. When sails are custom-cut for a boat, sailmakers add extra material and extra seams at chafe locations.

Sails arrive at their designed shape by the combination of various shapes that are sewn together. This sewing may be either by hand or by machine. "Hand-sewn" sails are the pride of the sailor; they are more expensive, but claimed to be longer lasting.

The overwhelming choice of sail on pleasure boats today is the triangular fore-and-aft Marconi. Its predecessors are the four-sided gaff sail and, further back in time, the square sail used so effectively by the clipper ships. the Marconi rig is high and comparatively narrow with a high aspect ratio (the ratio of the height to the width). The tip (head) of the Marconi is hoisted to the masthead, and the bottom edge (foot) is either bent on a boom or free (loose-footed). The forward edge of the sail (luff) is in tracks on the mast. The after edge of the triangular sail has pockets for the battens that are inserted to maintain the designed shape against the wind.

A sail may look "flat" to the casual observer, but actually it mimics an airplane wing when on the wind and thus supplies "lift." This lift is in a forward direction and translates into propulsion of the boat. The sail shape causes the wind to travel at different velocities over the front and back, with resulting "lift" in a forward direction. (The transformation of velocity into force is known as the Bernoulli effect.)

SAILS

The sailmaker builds shape into the sail by means of panels. The scientifically designed sail is composed of sewn-together sections in which the warp of the fabric may run in different directions in order to accommodate the "belly."

The "leech" and the "luff" are the sailor's way of designating the forward and after edges of the sail, respectively. A reinforcement built into the leech of the sail, called a "roach," helps maintain the aerodynamic action. Sails are also often "roped" for additional sturdiness, with a small-diameter line sewn all around the edge. Short lengths of line set at intervals above the foot of the sail are called "reef points" and provide a means of shortening the amount of sail exposed to the wind in heavy weather.

When the boat is running down wind, it is simply being pushed, and its speed cannot exceed that of the wind. A very large, light sail, known as a "spinnaker" and opening like an umbrella, takes full advantage of the wind when running downwind. Sailors run riot in their choice of wild colors when it comes to balloon spinnakers.

Maintenance Dacron sails require little maintenance beyond keeping them clean, shading them from the sun when not in use, and always being alert for seams about to let go. A thorough freshwater hosing is good medicine, especially after a run in salt water. Enough salt becomes encrusted on the sails to create a focus for trouble. Probably the weakest characteristic of Dacron is its vulnerability to the ultraviolet rays of the sun. When the sail is doused, it should go into a bag or else go below—unless roller-furling makes this precaution unnecessary.

The cringles (eyelets) at head, tack, and clew (the three corners) of the sail should be examined for corrosion and for their tightness in the cloth. Ditto for the mast track slides on the luff, and the boom track slides on the foot, in the case of a mainsail.

The wise skipper checks with his sailmaker at the first sign of sailwear. Delay is a poor economy, because the sail can only get worse.

Repair Repair jobs on the sail may consist of replacing seams, applying patches, and setting in new cringles. Do-it-yourself sewing is difficult, especially on the heavier weights of Dacron, but not impossible. Sewing kits, available at marine suppliers, contain needles, waxed Dacron thread, and the absolutely essential leather "palm." (The palm protects the sailor like a thimble does the dressmaker.)

Small tears may be repaired, without sewing, with adhesive patches, but at best this makes a temporary fix. A typical sewn repair requires a patch several inches larger than the tear and placed centrally over it. The tear is cut out to a small rectangle whose perimeter is sewn centrally to the patch. The perimeter of the patch is then closely stitched to the sail.

When it comes to cringles, metal hole protectors (they require a correct-size punch and die), and long seams, the work is best left to the sailmaker. Metal slides on the sail should be watched for corrosion that can stain the sail. (Note that most stain-removing procedures weaken the sail.)

Satellite Navigation Systems

Satellites, already common in many forms of electronic communication, now bring their advantages to the seven seas to provide super-accurate fixes for the passagemaking skipper. (A "fix," to a skipper, is any definitely located point on a chart.) Best of all, obtaining these fixes from knowledge of the satellite orbit requires only simple manipulation of a special receiver and almost no expertise. Logically, the satellite track is minutely known and becomes the reference from which the ship's position is derived.

The satellite navigation systems available today for working up a fix are: the Global Positioning System (GPS), the Sat-Nav System, and the Transit System. Of these, GPS is the newest and, in fact, is destined for completion only in the early 1990s, with a target date of Fall 1993, though it is already operable on most important world ocean runs. A typical GPS satellite orbits approximately 600 miles above the Earth at a velocity of approximately 275 miles per minute. The full-blown Global Positioning System is capable of such great positioning accuracy that the Defense Department fears it may become useful to an enemy. Accordingly, the system is purposely downgraded for civilian use. The completed GPS will include twenty-one satellites, of which three will be held in reserve. (At this writing there are thirteen operational.) A complete fix will require three satellites simultaneously, and these will be available around the clock.

The Transit System also is scheduled to add to the number of its new satellites; at present it has six in polar orbit. These satellites are under the control of a series of tracking and injection stations. The tracking stations constantly monitor minute changes in orbit due to gravity, and the injection stations store this information aboard the satellite for rebroadcast to ships seeking fixes. A complete encirclement of the Earth on the polar orbit takes 127 minutes, but the fact that all planned satellites are not yet in service may cause hours of delay for a ship seeking a fix.

At present writing, the Sat-Nav System is the most in use.

The first step in position finding is to locate the satellite's "closest point of approach" (CPA). This is accomplished by making use of the Doppler effect on the 400-megahertz working radio frequency, an automatic function of the receiver (see Doppler Effect). The satellite now rebroadcasts the positioning data sent to it by the injection station. The skipper feeds in some requested dead-reckoning (DR) numbers into the receiver, and presto! a fix.

Dead reckoning entails keeping exact records of speed, direction, and time and vectoring these into a result that may be charted as a fix; see Vectors. The (DR) numbers are the speed, the heading, the latitude and longitude, GMT (Greenwich Mean Time), and the height of the receiving antenna.

The request for antenna height is unusual and needs explanation. At the instant of CPA, the satellite is still at orbital height and its angle with the receiving antenna may vary widely, from that with a small boat to that with an ocean liner. This variation affects the accuracy of the final fix.

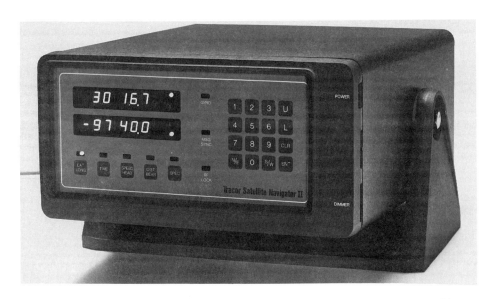

SATELLITE NAVIGATION SYSTEMS—This marvel of modern electronics receives information from satellites and automatically processes it into a highly accurate fix. *(Courtesy Magellan)*

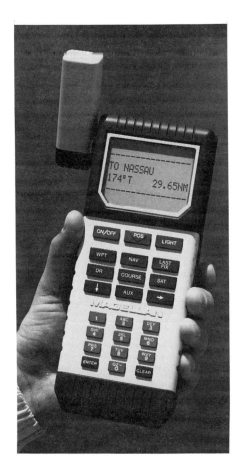

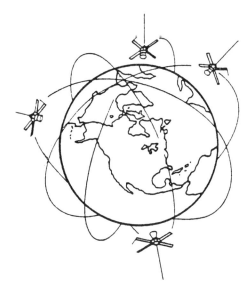

SATELLITE NAVIGATION SYSTEMS—This instrument establishes a vessel's position by computations combining the data broadcast by the passing satellite with the Doppler effect plus boat speed and heading. Pilot lights announce the lock-on to the satellite broadcast and the reception of the data. *(Courtesy Tracor Inc.)*

SEA ANCHORS

The receivers are designed for extremely high frequency at which a piece of wire has inductance without being coiled.

The high radio frequency (approximately 400 megahertz) mandates a short whip antenna that may be deteriorated by spray and salt. Consequently, the antenna is housed in a cylindrical, dome-end plastic container; plastic filling prevents vibration. These cylinders are often seen today on the highest locations on large ships. (See Antennas.)

There is a difference in operational result between this satellite navigation system and Loran. Loran provides continuous readings of position, while the satellite may cause hours of waiting. An obvious panacea is to have both systems aboard for serious passagemaking.

Of the DR numbers that must be plugged into the receiver, an error in speed has a predictable result on the accuracy of the final fix. The fix will have an error of two-tenths of a mile for each knot of error in speed. The DR numbers mentioned above may be added to the receiver manually, but on most big-ship installations the additions take place automatically. Some form of log keeps continuous count on vessel speed. The latitude/longitude may be the skipper's calculation of position or the reading from a Loran. The GMT (Greenwich Mean time) is readily available from worldwide radio time transmissions.

Certain satellite combinations may result in doubtful readings, but this generally is self-apparent. This is similar to the case where two LOPs (lines of position; see Direction Finders) meet at an angle too sharp for accuracy. The sharper the angle, the more it approximates the point of an arrow.

The latest designs of GPS receivers are portable, small enough to be hand held, and accept input such as speed and heading from other instruments.

Installation and service of this equipment should be by professionals.

Sea Anchors

A sea anchor is a rewarding piece of equipment for a rough-water, offshore skipper. Whether store-bought or home-made, a sea anchor can make life aboard a bit more comfortable while riding out a severe blow.

The conventional sea anchor is a large fabric cone held to its open shape by metal or plastic hoops. A tow line is attached to shrouds at the circular open end of the cone. A trip line attaches to the apex. The construction usually is collapsible to facilitate storage. (Luckily, storms wild enough to call for the sea anchor do not occur often.)

Since a sea anchor spends most of its life in a locker, it is wise to choose one made of synthetic fabric that does not rot.

The sea anchor is set from the bow with the boat pointing into the wind and sea. The drag that results keeps the bow from falling off to one side and the other, so that the boat takes the storm head-on, rather than beam-to. This does not stop the boat firmly as a reg-

SEACOCKS

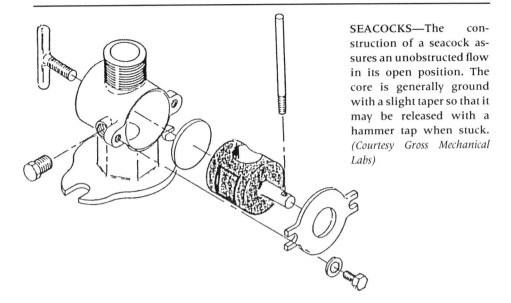

SEACOCKS—The construction of a seacock assures an unobstructed flow in its open position. The core is generally ground with a slight taper so that it may be released with a hammer tap when stuck. *(Courtesy Gross Mechanical Labs)*

ular anchor would, but allows it to drift. This drift naturally is to leeward, and any shoals in that direction must be guarded against, if possible, with a true anchor.

When the danger is over, the sea anchor is hauled aboard with the trip line. This moves the sea anchor through the water point-first, with minimum resistance.

The sea anchor may also be used as a "drogue," this time from the stern. The occasion for this is a following sea and wind that try to swing the stern around into a broach. The drag of the drogue keeps the stern plumb with the bow. The action is most effective when some way (forward motion) is kept on.

Some sea anchors make provision for an oil bag to smooth the waves. A small amount of oil is sufficient for this purpose because the oil spreads out until the film is only one molecule thick. It is a matter of surface tension. (The monomolecular nature of the film is the reason for the rainbow colors.)

Seacocks

A seacock is a special valve designed to control the flow of intake or exhaust water at a through-hull opening below the waterline. The preferred material is bronze, with emphasis on alloys having minimal loss of zinc through internal chemical action.

The seacock is generally flanged at one end and is left as a plain pipe to take hose at the other. The flange is bolted over the inside of the through-hull opening, usually with a companion flange on the outside. One end of the seacock's rotatable core is squared to fit a removable handle, while the other end has a threaded extension for a nut.

The core and the mating internal surface of the seacock are ground to a slight taper. This is ingenious, because it prevents the core from ever becoming irremovably jammed. Were the core to resist turning, a light hammer tap would release it. Open and closed

SEAGOING CLOCKS

Half hour	1 bell	ding			
1 hour	2 bells	ding-ding			
1½ hours	3 bells	ding-ding,	ding		
2 hours	4 bells	ding-ding,	ding-ding		
2½	5 bells	ding-ding,	ding-ding,	ding	
3 hours	6 bells	ding-ding,	ding-ding,	ding-ding	
3½ hours	7 bells	ding-ding,	ding-ding,	ding-ding,	ding
4 hours	8 bells	ding-ding,	ding-ding,	ding-ding,	ding-ding
Repeat					

seacocks are distinguished from each other by a 90-degree turn, thus making handle position a reliable indicator.

A screen commonly covers the outside opening to keep out nosy fish.

Installation Seacocks should be located where hull strength is sufficient to resist the side thrusts caused by operating them. Hoses attached to seacocks should be double-clamped. The core of a seacock should be coated very lightly with marine grease before installation.

Troubleshooting If reasonable force on the handle fails to turn a seacock open or shut, the following procedure should be followed: Loosen the nut and unscrew it until it extends just beyond its threaded stud. Tap the nut (*not* the stud) with a hammer; this protects the threads.

ing a crew member on guard. While en route, each watch was of four hours' duration. The ding-dings are matched to a four-hour span.

Everything starts at midnight (1200 hours), continues for four hours, and repeats, with a single ding added for each half hour. Thus, 12:30, the first half hour of the night watch, is marked by one ding. One o'clock adds a ding, to make the sounding "ding-ding." But the next half hour does not get three dings in a row; instead, the clock sounds "ding-ding, ding."

Maintenance Most of these seagoing clocks run one week on a winding, and it improves accuracy if they are wound at regular weekly intervals—for instance, every Sunday morning. Some of these clocks are run by flashlight cells and require no attention for months.

Seagoing Clocks

The "ding-ding" of seagoing clocks puzzles the landlubber—and many a new skipper, too. Yet it is a simple system that grew out of the method of maintaining four-hour watches keep-

Self-Steerers

Taking the helm of a sailboat is romantic and fun–unless the trick at the

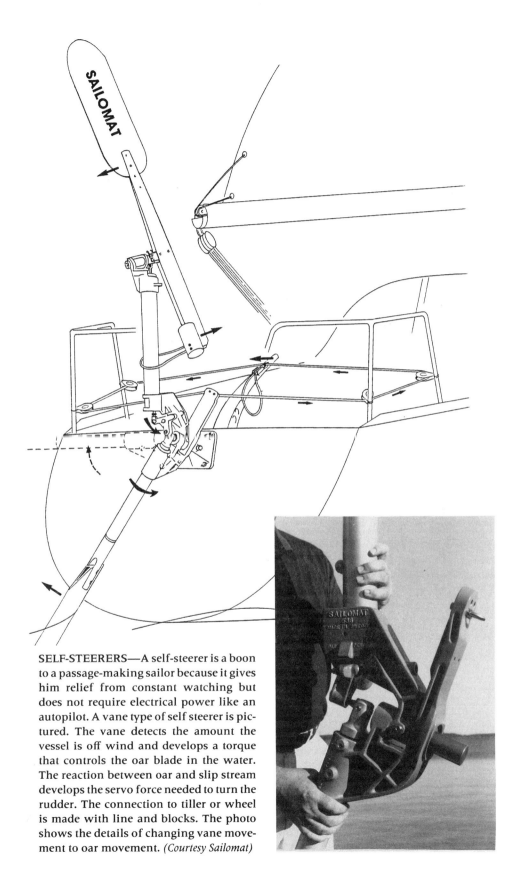

SELF-STEERERS—A self-steerer is a boon to a passage-making sailor because it gives him relief from constant watching but does not require electrical power like an autopilot. A vane type of self steerer is pictured. The vane detects the amount the vessel is off wind and develops a torque that controls the oar blade in the water. The reaction between oar and slip stream develops the servo force needed to turn the rudder. The connection to tiller or wheel is made with line and blocks. The photo shows the details of changing vane movement to oar movement. *(Courtesy Sailomat)*

wheel or tiller extends into the weary hours. Then boredom may take over, and even a born sailor may think of forswearing sailing. One relief on a long passage is a mechanical steerer that needs no outside power.

The self-steerer is rigged on the stern of the sailboat. It consists of a system of vanes and levers to control the rudder with a preset relationship to the wind. What takes place is a form of "servo" action.

A vertical vane, supported in a bearing to swing horizontally, reacts to the apparent wind and attempts to align itself parallel to it. The movement of this vane is transmitted to a small servo rudder that uses the energy in the stream of water to move the main rudder that steers the boat. If the boat veers off course, counter-forces are generated to bring it back.

Before fitting a boat with self-steering, the skipper must make sure the boat itself is amenable to self-steering. This takes into account such characteristics as waterline/beam ratios, keel lengths, sail plan, range of center-of-effort location. Roughly summarized, self-steering is most successful with sailboats that like to stay on course, at least on most headings.

Frankly stated, mechanical steerers cannot display the accuracy of holding course of which electric and hydraulic autopilots are capable. But self-steerers can transform the continuous attention required at the helm into periods of supervision that are much less tiring.

Maintenance The many linkages and bearings of a self-steerer must be kept lubricated and free. Repeated reference to the compass should verify the action of the self-steerer. It seems that the self-steerer relies for accuracy as much on the skipper's expert hand as on itself. Since the parts of a self-steerer are all in the open, troubleshooting and repair become a matter of observation and commonsense.

Shore Cables

The shore-power cable feeds electric current from the marina mains to the boat tied up alongside. Standardization of cable end connectors and of shore-side outlets makes it possible for a boat to plug in routinely at any marina for instant power. Shore-power cables are available in either of two ratings, 30 ampere or 50 ampere, and 25 feet or 50 feet long, in three-wire or four-wire makeup (see Wiring Color Code).

Heavy individual wire insulations are covered overall with a thick plastic abrasion-resistant layer that protects against the inevitable scraping along the pier. (With incorrect slack, the shore cable often functions as an unintended intermittent dock line.)

The cruising skipper should carry cable adapters that enable his shore cable to function with the various outlets found on marina piers.

Multiplying the cable's ampere rating by the alternating-current voltage gives a rough approximation of the amount of power, in watts, that may safely be brought from shore. This is then matched with the sum of the individual powers, in watts, needed aboard.

SINGLE SIDEBAND

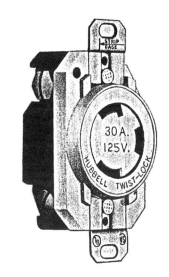

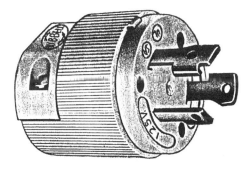

SHORE CABLES—The end fittings on shore cables determine the maximum current for which they are designed. Differences in the blade pattern prevent interconnecting differently rated cables. *(Courtesy Hubbell)*

Troubleshooting A warm-to-the-touch shore cable is a warning of overload; only the barest hint of warmth is within limits. The shore cable should be so arranged at its terminals as to prevent tensile stress to the inlet and outlet fittings to which it attaches.

Repair An accidentally parted shore cable may be spliced, but this had better be done professionally with copper cable clamps and approved insulating materials. Most likely, the repaired area no longer will be truly waterproof.

Single Sideband

For radio communication beyond the nominal 25-mile range of the VHF transceiver, the pleasure-boat skipper has available a more powerful style of transmission called "single sideband" (SSB). SSB is legally allotted more power than VHF, and it uses that power more effectively.

SSB is an amplitude-modulated (AM) system, and, as such, its waveform has three parts: a lower sideband, a carrier, and an upper sideband. The uniqueness of SSB arises when the carrier and one sideband are removed before transmission and the total power is concentrated in that one remaining sideband. The result is a transmission containing almost eight times the power of the equivalent AM.

The Federal Communications Commission designates the transmission of only the one sideband as "A3J." One sideband with the carrier is "A3H." One sideband with reduced carrier is "A3A."

Standard AM receivers cannot receive the A3J transmissions. For this reason, all SSB installations are legally required to be able to transmit in A3H style on the 2,182-kilohertz distress frequency. Automatic distress alarms at the Coast Guard and on commercial

SINGLE SIDEBAND

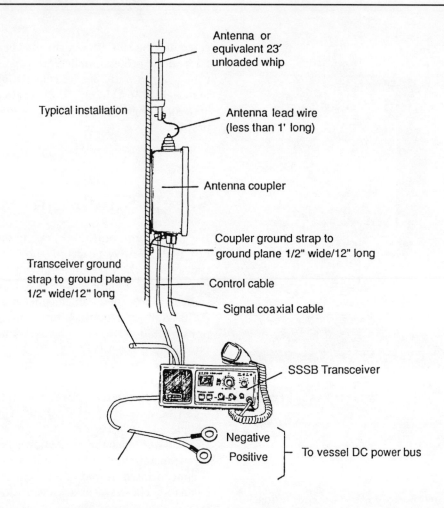

Typical installation

SINGLE SIDEBAND—Cautions for installation: The antenna coupler must be less than 1 foot from the antenna, and the ground connections must be "perfect." In the late SSB models, the coupler automatically tunes the antennas to the receiver and transmitter selected frequencies. The July, 1991, upheaval in single sideband frequency allocations affects every SSB user. Every SSB transceiver must be realigned by a licensed technician.

ships stand by continuously for possible SOS signals.

SSB communication is restricted to a number of channels in the radio spectrum between 2 megahertz and 23 megahertz. For efficient energy transfer over this entire wide frequency span, the antenna must be tunable to each point of operation. This tuning is accomplished by an antenna coupler situated directly below the antenna; this action is automatic (see Antennas).

The need for tuning the antenna to

resonance (exactly identical frequency) at the frequency being used exists not only to assure the maximum transfer of energy. The resonance also protects the transmitter from unradiated energy that otherwise would be reflected back. The degree of success in directing all the transmitter energy into the antenna is expressed by the "voltage standing wave ratio" (VSWR). A VSWR of 1 to 1 is an unattainable ideal; up to 1 to 2 is tolerable. (See Standing Wave Ratio.)

The propagation of radio waves at the frequencies used for SSB is affected by planetary and weather conditions. Thus, the condition of the ionosphere, a reflective shell enclosing the Earth, governs the choice of the most effective frequency for a given transmission, and such knowledge becomes part of an operator's expertise.

Whereas the VHF transceiver is held to a maximum power of 25 watts, the SSB transceiver is available with six times this power. The result is long-range communicating ability, suitable even for a passagemaker

Installation The connection between antenna and antenna coupler is critical and should be a short copper strap. The ground connection to the coupler is equally critical and should run directly to the ship's main ground (see Grounds). The transceiver itself also needs good grounding; a bad ground here may make the operator part of the radiation system.

Maintenance The only maintenance on an SSB within the capability of the skipper is to maintain general cleanliness, dryness, and constant inspection of all ground connections for corrosion. Adjustments must be made by a licensed technician.

Soldering

Whenever two or more wires must be connected together for the efficient passage of electric current, soldering is the preferred method. A properly soldered connection becomes homogeneous metal with a reasonable chance of surviving the marine environment. (It's true that telephone companies, with their millions of connections, have abandoned soldering. But they have substituted a wire-winding technique in which one wire actually cuts into the other to achieve good contact.)

In the soldering process, a metal with low melting point (the solder) is heated, melted, and caused to attach itself to the wires that are to be joined. On cooling of the solder, the wires and any connector become one.

The secret of expert soldering lies in two words: cleanliness and heat. The wires, the soldering iron, and the connectors must be not just kitchen clean but chemically clean. All the surfaces must be abraded down to shiny base metal as a preliminary step. This is done with abrasive paper or, on corroded surfaces, with a fine file. Subsequent fingerprinting is avoided. The soldering iron must be able to maintain a temperature higher than the solder's melting point. However, to prevent heat from harming delicate components, a "heat sink" may be used, such as the long-nosed pliers shown in the diagram (see Heat Sinks).

The solder is an alloy of lead and tin. It is supplied as a miniature tubing filled with "flux." The flux is a rosin that melts over the area to be soldered and prevents obstructive oxidation. The commercial name of this solder is

SOLDERING

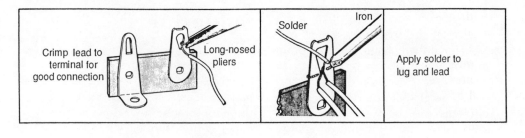

SOLDERING—Some bad is always mixing in with the good, even in soldering. Plenty of heat is good for soldering—but it may be bad for delicate components. A simple scheme for protection is shown in the drawings. A pair of pliers is used as a heat sink.

"rosin core solder," and it is the only kind used in electrical work; "acid core solder" is *never* used.

The first step in a soldering job is to "tin" the soldering iron. The iron is brought to working temperature, and its tip is touched with the solder. Assuming the iron is at the correct temperature, its entire tip should immediately be covered with solder through capillary attraction. (Note that this is the *only* time during the soldering operation that solder is presented directly to the iron, because re-tinning should not become necessary.)

With the wires in place, the tip of the soldering iron is now held to them to bring them quickly up to soldering temperature. The solder is then touched to the wires and allowed to melt over them. Capillarity will cause the solder to cover the bare metal surfaces. A silver, mirror-like appearance of the melted solder at this stage of the operation is an indication of good workmanship. (A dull solder flow is known in the trade as a "pasted connection." This is a sign of insufficient heat and is certain to cause eventual trouble if allowed to remain.) By the way, the wires must be kept motionless while the melted solder is solidifying.

When everything has cooled down, the flux will have become hard and cracked and easy to remove, if desired.

At cleanup time, the soldering iron may be hastened in its cooling by holding the tip in cold water—but *only* the tip.

The market offers soldering irons in many sizes and styles. The ability of the iron to generate heat is expressed in wattage. The higher the rated watts, the heavier the work that may be undertaken. One pound and heavier coppers are heated in braziers and are used by tinsmiths. Light coppers, weighing in at a few ounces, solder the intricate connections of miniature circuit boards.

Interestingly, the many run-of-the-mill connections that comprise a circuit board are not made with soldering irons. They are made simultaneously by an ingenious method: The circuit board, with all its units in place, is floated on the melted surface of a tank of solder. Capillarity brings the solder to every planned connection and bonds it. A painted or printed resistive coating keeps the solder from going to forbidden areas.

Most soldering irons are not temperature controlled; their temperature depends largely on the amount of time they are plugged in. However, soldering-iron stands are available that provide temperature control for the iron placed on them.

Repair There are occasions when solder must be *removed* from connections, as when repairing electronic circuit boards. A tool designed for this purpose is available in the radio shops. It is a small soldering iron with a suction tube next to the tip; pressing a rubber bulb provides the suction.

The solder on the connection to be removed is melted with the iron. The melted solder is sucked up with a few squeezes of the bulb.

Spark Plugs

The spark plug's simplicity of construction belies its importance in the functioning of internal combustion engines. The spark plug ignites the fuel in the cylinder and begins the conversion of energy into work.

The spark plug consists of a steel tube, threaded to fit the engine location, containing a central ceramic insulator. An electrode runs through the insulator to form a threaded connection at the top, and a gap with an extension from the steel tube at the bottom. The assembly is gas-tight.

When the spark plug is screwed into the engine to its complete depth it makes a gas-tight seal. In some spark plugs this sealing is accomplished with a gasket; in others with an accurately machined taper that matches the engine taper. The "heat range" for which the spark plug is useful is determined by how far the "nose" of the insulator projects from the body, the longer the nose the hotter the plug's "heat range" rating.

The spark plug insulator must be immune to great thermal shock. Within minutes after the engine is first started, the spark plug is seared by blast furnace flame, so it must be immune to great thermal shock. It must not develop hot spots that could cause preignition. Naturally the insulator must resist the approximately 50,000 volts delivered by modern ignition systems.

The gap where the spark takes place is adjustable by careful bending. The length of this gap must match the ignitability of the fuel. For many years .035" was a quasi standard. Modern engines have leaner fuel mixtures so they generally require a lengthening of the gap to .050".

Most of today's automotive spark plugs contain an internal resistor. This is added to prevent interference with surrounding radio reception. (Each

SPARK PLUGS

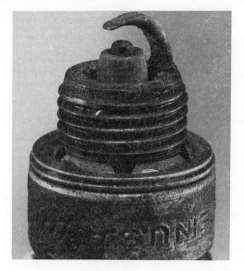
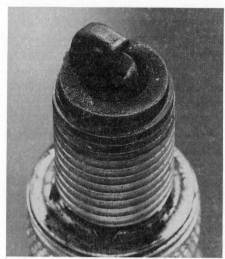
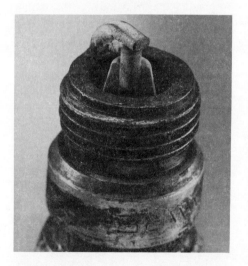
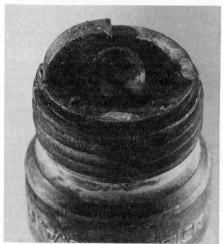

SPARK PLUGS—A close inspection of the business end of spark plugs can reveal much about the internal condition of the engine. The results of four common engine ailments are shown here. At A, a worn out plug. At B, a carbon-fouled plug. At C, the result of detonation. At D, what preignition does. *(Courtesy Spark Plug Co.)*

spark generates an offending radio wave that is aborted by the resistor.)

Spark plugs are manufactured to fit hundreds of different specifications. Only one particular plug is correct for a given engine. It is identified by Part Number in the Owner's Manual.

Spark plug maintenance begins with correct installation. The plug should be inserted and run to its thread end by hand. Then a correct size socket wrench should be used to tighten it to the remaining partial turn. Modern ignition cables contain resistance material (to further check radio interference) and must be handled with care, never "yanked". The ceramic insulator should be kept clean, as should the hollow in the engine.

An inspection of the spark plugs can reveal a lot about the operating condition of the engine. Four common examples are shown by the photographs. At A is a plug that is simply worn out. The spark has eroded the gap terminal. The voltage required for a spark is now so high that it endangers the coil. At B is a plug that has been carbon fouled. The insulator is covered with a soft black sooty deposit that acts as an easier path for the voltage than the gap, hence no spark. At C is an example of detonation. The undesired shock wave that detonation causes has fractured the insulator nose. (One cause of detonation is too low an octane rating of the fuel.) At D is shown one result of preignition. The gap terminals have been partially melted away by the excess heat. (Glowing carbon deposits in a dirty engine will cause preignition.)

Worn or damaged spark plugs are discarded. Fouled plugs may be cleaned with the aid of a narrow scraper. Gap lengths are set with available simple gauges. The correct gap opening is determined from the Owner's Manual.

Spring Lines

Spring lines are a skipper's best friend and helper. Spring lines are used to help spot the boat into difficult pier positions. Spring lines check the lateral movement of the boat along the pier, important when a gangway is rigged or other vessels are close by. (Intrinsically, the spring line is not different from the other lines aboard; it differs only in its use.)

Four spring lines are in common usage: the forward bow spring, the after bow spring, the forward quarter spring, the after quarter spring. The bow springs run from a chock and cleat slightly aft of the bow, the quarter springs from a chock and cleat just forward of the stern (known as "the quarter"). Rarely, a boat will have a chock and cleat at the most useful spot of all, at center length. (Both sides of the boat are identically chocked and cleated.) The center position adds the choice of two additional springs.

The spring line functions in maneuvering a boat by being the fixed-length tension-link in a system comprising the rudder, the power, and the resistance of wind or current. When holding a boat closely to a given spot, the spring lines simply become tight reins. The actual stresses of remaining

Stabilizers

The sea and the human stomach have always been at odds, and a storm may drive even a veteran sailor to lean over the rail. Stabilizers to iron out the sickening roll consequently are either an installed feature on passagemaking ships or a desired accessory.

Stabilizers function by generating a force equal and opposite to that of the roll. Thus, theoretically at least, the roll is canceled out and the hull is not deflected. The negation of rolling is counted on as well to reduce yawing and pitching, motions that also affect comfort.

Stabilizers require a sensor to alert them to rolling conditions and to synchronize the counter-efforts. Such sensors have various degrees of complexity and sensitivity. Among the most effective are gyroscopes because of their natural tendency to maintain a fixed alignment with space when they are spinning. They maintain an artificial vertical against which the roll is compared and by which the necessary counter-action is released. The gyro is driven electrically, mechanically, or hydraulically.

The design of stabilizers varies with the manufacturer. Some stabilizers use two active surfaces, some four. Some stabilizer elements are rotating surfaces. How these surfaces move also varies. All attempt to meet each roll with opposite and equal force.

The reactive force to stop the roll is exerted against the water by planes or fins. The fins are shaped to give aerodynamic "lift" and thereby increase their effectiveness.

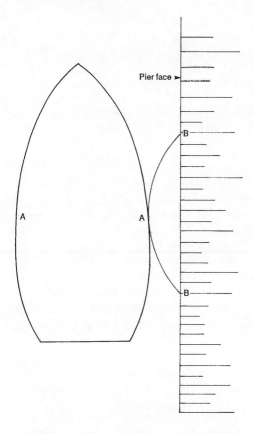

SPRING LINES—Shown is a simple spring line pattern that prevents a boat from "walking" back and forth along a pier. At A are a chock and a cleat. At B is a cleat or a pile. The slack in the line depends upon tidal conditions. (Bow and stern lines also will be set.)

docked are assumed by the bow and stern lines. Note that a forward line *runs* forward, and an after line *runs* aft. Lines at right angle to boat length are "breast" lines and may be used at the bow and the stern.

STABILIZERS

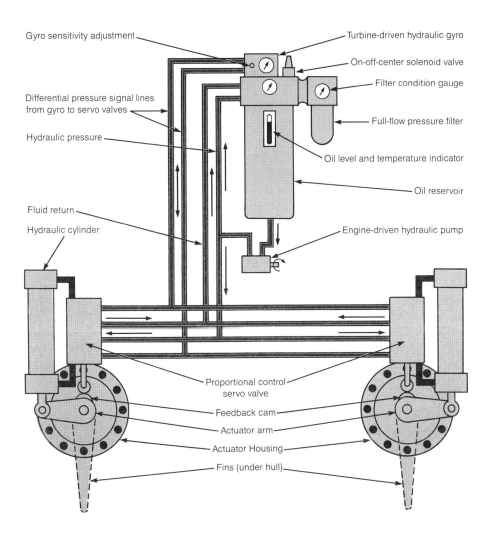

STABILIZERS—The manner in which a hydraulically operated stabilizer is interconnected is shown, together with photos of the individual parts. *(Courtesy Naiad)*

STANDING WAVE RATIO

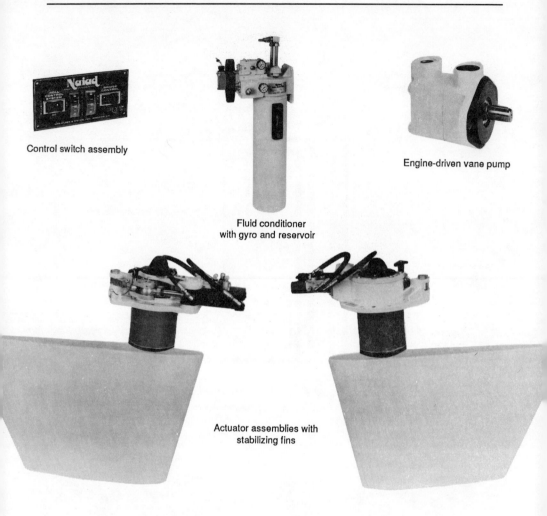

Control switch assembly

Fluid conditioner with gyro and reservoir

Engine-driven vane pump

Actuator assemblies with stabilizing fins

The power needed to overcome rolling is generally taken from the propulsion engine, without any decrease in boat performance. The manufacturers claim that stabilizers are applicable to boats as small as 38 feet overall.

One should not lose sight of the fact that the use of stabilizers imposes a great stress upon the hull. Destructive forces appear that are far greater than any imposed by merely rolling in a sea. Careful appraisal of hull strength is necessary.

Standing Wave Ratio

The fact that the radio transmitter develops 25 watts does not necessarily mean that this full amount of power reaches the antenna. Actually, there are losses, and these will be considerable if the transmission line and the antenna are not "matched." The losses are technically expressed as "standing wave ratio" (SWR). By definition, the

STANDING WAVE RATIO

SWR is the ratio of the transmission line "characteristic impedance" to the characteristic impedance of the antenna. (Impedance is the alternating-current counterpart of direct-current resistance.)

Ideally, the impedances would be equal and the SWR would be 1 to 1—a condition not practically attainable because of unavoidable power loss. An SWR of 2 to 1 is considered desirable.

When the impedances of transmission line and antenna input are equal, waves traveling down the line do not realize the end of the line and make a smooth, loss-less crossover. With inequality, some of the waves are bounced back to the transmitter. The presence in the line of waves moving in both directions breeds the "standing waves." The reflected waves may be harmful to the transmitter.

While all this may sound complicated, a simple procedure is open to the skipper. Standing wave meters are available at moderate cost. These meters give direct readings. Installation consists of simply coupling the meters into the transmission line with standard connectors. The SWR meter gives a reading of transmitter efficiency every time the push-to-talk button is pressed.

Most manufacturers supply a 25-watt SWR meter to go with VHF transceivers. (See VHF-FM Radio.)

Starters

The starter motor cranks the propulsion engine in response to the turn of a key or the push of a button on the remote console. This series-wound, high-torque, high-current motor meshes its pinion gear with the flywheel ring gear when a start is demanded and turns the engine over at proper cranking speed. The current drawn from the battery to do this usually is in the hundreds of amperes.

The required mesh of pinion gear and ring gear is accomplished in one of several methods, depending upon design: (A), a spiral-grooved shaft forces the pinion forward when the starter motor acquires speed; (B), a solenoid advances the pinion when current is applied; (C), the entire armature (rotor) is pushed outward magnetically. The teeth of both pinion and of ring gear are shaped to accommodate this sliding mesh.

After the few seconds it takes to get the engine going, the gears must be unmeshed. This is necessary because the extreme ratio between the huge ring gear and the diminutive pinion would spin the starter motor to complete wreckage. Springs, the deactivation of the solenoid, the spiral shaft, and an over-running clutch are all concerned with setting the starter motor back to rest. The starter motor simply stands by when the engine is running.

The torque required of the starter motor determines whether it is wound with heavy copper wire or with copper strip, the latter being chosen for the heavier duty. The armature (rotor) winding connects with the bars of the commutator in a strict pattern. The field (stator) winding is distributed over the two, four, or six poles the design entails. The armature turns concentrically within the field poles. The

STARTERS

series form of winding provides the highest torque, and consequently the starter motor is internally connected in this mode. (see Electricity)

The heavy current in the starter system makes a large contact relay necessary. The solenoid combines such a relay with its job of moving the pinion into mesh. When the solenoid plunger is drawn forward by actuation of the solenoid winding, it closes the contacts and meshes the pinion simultaneously.

Most propulsion engines still follow the automotive style of placing the starter at the bottom of the flywheel. This is fine for cars because it makes the starter easily accessible from underneath. For boats, this style does the opposite: It puts the starter motor down into the bilge where it is hard to get at. Furthermore, the unit is at a low level where dangerous fuel fumes could collect and be ignited by a spark. Because of this danger, starters in this position are subject to a safety rule requiring solid covers over all contacts.

Maintenance The starter motor is in use for only a small fraction of the running time of the engine, and its maintenance needs are almost none. Starter cable connections should be kept to bright metal, and the wires should not be able to immerse themselves in the bilge. Insulation that is noticeably giving way should be thoroughly bound with electrical-grade tape. Generally there is no provision for oiling, but a few drops on the pinion are worthwhile.

Troubleshooting Troubleshooting logic: The wiring comprises a low-current circuit from the starter key to the solenoid and a high-current circuit between the battery and the starter motor.

Key is turned, starter does not respond: Each turn of the key should elicit a click from the solenoid or relay. If there is no click, check wiring from key switch. If click is evident, but starter does not turn (battery assumed good), check for corroded terminal connections. If key sets starter motor spinning fast but not cranking, pinion is not meshing, either because it is stuck on its spiral or because of faulty mechanical connection between solenoid plunger and pinion assembly.

Key is turned, starter stalls: Battery is too low, or cable connection is corroded and causing excessive voltage drop. (Sometimes a low battery causes a series of clicks as the starter keeps trying.)

A simple check to determine approximate battery condition: Keep a light bulb turned on while actuating the starter. The light should dim only moderately, not excessively. An actual voltage reading may be obtained with the VOM in the voltmeter mode by having the meter leads attached to the battery while the starter is turned on (see Voltohmmeter, Volt-and-ampere meters). The reading should not fall below 9 volts.

It is a foregone conclusion that in a marine atmosphere, most of the troubles encountered may be placed at the door of corrosion.

Repair The high cost of labor makes it impractical to repair a given starter motor. The normal procedure is to take it to an automotive electric shop and exchange it for a "rebuilt" unit that is "as good as new."

Static

Static was the bane of all radio communication until the invention of frequency modulation (FM) freed that system from the clicks, whistles, and bangs. But amplitude modulation (AM) remains vulnerable to this day.

Static exists as man-made interference or as the result of electrical dis-

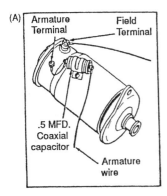

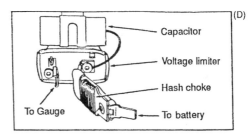

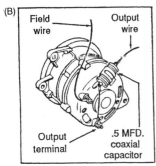

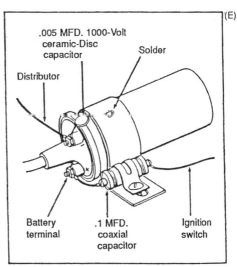

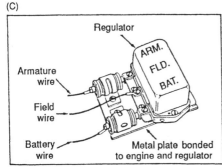

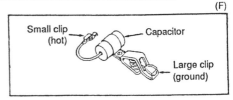

STATIC—The capacitors shunt radio interference (man-made static) to ground and prevent detriment to radio communications. Note that field (control) wires are not broken for capacitor insertion. *(Courtesy Champion Spark Plug)*

163

STEERING TORQUE

charges taking place naturally all over the Earth. The saving grace is that the man-made noises may be prevented, while the natural ones may not. Modern circuit design and construction have been a great help in getting the message through despite Nature's objection.

Anything aboard that requires electric current to be turned on and off can be the source of static. Luckily, this form of man-made static is easily killed at the source, as shown in the drawings. The capacitors form a low-resistance short for any spark and prevent the radio wave from radiating.

Coaxial capacitors are best for this noise-reducing service (see Capacitors). Where they are to carry current, as for an output, they must be specified to bear the intended load. Connections must be as close to zero resistance as possible. Note that the control wire, the field wire on generators and alternators, is not cut for a capacitor.

Capacitors may be tested for good or bad with a voltohmmeter (see Voltohmmeter). Resistance of a good capacitor should be infinite. A slight tick of the needle should take place on connection. A reverse tick should accompany reversing the connections.

Steering Torque

The effort required to turn the steering wheel and activate the entire steering system, including the rudder is called "steering torque." This rotative effort is expressed as "pound-feet." Note the difference from straight-line work that is rated in foot-pounds.

Mathematically, torque equals the radius of the wheel, in feet or inches, multiplied by the force, in pounds, applied at the rim. Thus, a force of 1 pound at the rim of a 2-foot-*diameter* wheel becomes 1 pound-foot. The formula holds equally true if inches and ounces are used, and the answer becomes "ounce-inches."

An exact knowledge of the steering torque requirement of the boat becomes important when an automatic pilot (autopilot) is to be added (see Autopilots). The motor in the pilot (or the

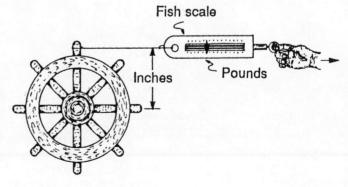

STEERING TORQUE—A common fish scale is rigged as shown in order to determine the number of pound-feet of torque the autopilot must supply to steer any given boat.

pump in a hydraulic system) obviously must have a torque rating greater than the requirement of the boat.

With automatic pilots that steer by moving the tiller, the situation is slightly different. The distance from the rudderpost to the point of application of the pilot to the tiller becomes the "radius" in the formula.

As with all adaptations of power to formerly manual tasks, the relative sizes must remain within certain limits. Too weak an autopilot will cause failure, too strong may result in jerky operation.

The neutral/forward/reverse mechanism is simple in the extreme: The sliding clutch dog is placed between two facing bevel gears that are driven by a bevel pinion on the vertical shaft. Thus, the dog may grip on to either gear for turning in either direction—or it may remain halfway between, out of contact, for neutral. These actions take place in response to the console control. Shifting of gears is facilitated by a trick commonly used on automobiles: The engine ignition is automatically killed for a fraction of a second at the instant of change. This momentar-

Stern-Drives

The stern-drive is an improvement over the outboard motor. It retains the advantages of the outboard motor but allows the use of a standard engine located inboard. The result is good control of the vessel, plus fuel economy. A bonus is an engine in a "get-at-able" location.

The stern-drive consists of a housing resembling the familiar outboard motor shape. This housing is in two parts. The upper half contains a horizontal shaft that goes to the engine. The lower half has the horizontal shaft to the propeller. A vertical shaft connects the two through the medium of bevel gears, and also has a pump that supplies cooling water to the engine. A universal joint is in the upper shaft line to the power plant. (See Universal Joints.) A clutch and dog on the lower shaft provide neutral, forward, and reverse.

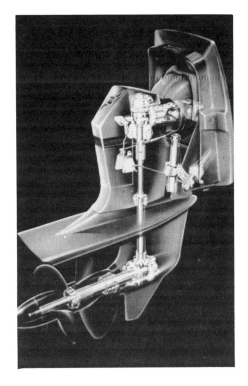

STERN-DRIVERS—This X-ray view shows the internal construction of a popular stern-drive. *(Courtesy Volvo Penta)*

STERN-DRIVES

ily relieves the drive system of torque and lets the clutch dog work smoothly.

The console control rods and Bowden wires also activate an important safety feature that prevents starting the engine unless the clutch is in neutral position (See Bowden Wires). This is accomplished by a switch in the ground line to the ignition coil. This switch is closed during forward and during reverse, but cuts the ground connection when the clutch is in the neutral mode. Without the coil ground, the ignition is dead.

The stern-drive unit is attached to and is supported by the transom of the boat. This means that not only is the transom loaded by the weight of the stern-drive, but it is subject to the reactions from the various torque forces generated underway. Obviously, a well-built, sturdy transom is number one on the list.

Installation The actual attachment to the transom is made via a bell housing, a gimbal ring, and a gimbal housing. The bell housing becomes part of the unit. The gimbal ring is firmly bolted to the transom. Visualize a universal joint for an explanation of the action between the two. The gimbal ring permits up-and-down (tilt) movement that regulates the angle of attack of the propeller against the water. The gimbal housing supplies right-and-left turning for steering. The available up-tilt is high enough to get the prop out of harm's way when the boat is being trailered. (Special hooks are available for locking the stern-drive firmly in the extra-high position.) (See Tilt/Trim.)

Pass-through holes are provided for cooling water; throttle, choke, clutch, and tilt cables; and engine exhaust. The final disposal of the exhaust is through the propeller hub, an easy way to reduce fumes and noise. The transition from fixed to movable pipe is made with bellows hose held firmly in place with cement and clamps. Senders on the stern-drive transmit a continuous position report to gauges on the console. The buttons for "up" and "down" also are on the console.

Maintenance Maintenance of the stern-drive concerns itself with lubrication and with observation of the stern-drive "unit." The lower portion of the drive unit has two lube holes covered by screws. The lower hole is the fill hole, the upper one the vent hole. The lubricant is forced into the lower hole until it appears at the upper hole to signal "full." The viscosity of this lube is too great to permit simple filling by gravity from the upper hole. Of course, the lubricants are those permitted by the owner's manual. (See Lubricating Oils.)

The steering wheel should be turned from hard-over (all the way) right to hard-over left in order to keep the cable lubricant distributed and the system limber. The owner's manual of a particular model is the source of specific instructions. Slightly more difficult is visual inspection of the bellows hoses and their clamps; laxity here could bring leaks.

Note the water-intake ports on the lower portion of the stern-drive, and never run the engine without these being fully immersed. Dry running will kill the impeller of the stern-drive water pump that always turns with the vertical shaft. (Water from flushing attachments can substitute for immersion.)

The propeller should feel solidly locked to the clutch when an attempt

STOVES

is made to hand-turn it after shifting into forward or reverse *with engine stopped* and ignition disabled. If this is not true, examine the shift cable and the system of shift rods. Examine the position and opening of the neutral switch.

Troubleshooting Troubleshooting logic: (The engine is assumed to be in running order; the concern is with the stern-drive only.) The stern-drive is a simple mechanical device, and any misfunction should be easily apparent.

Shifts into either forward or reverse, but not into both: Worn or disfigured bevel gear. Burr on horizontal shaft where dog clutch slides. Shift cable and rods not in synchronism. Damaged shift assembly in stern-drive.

Unusual running noises: Engine too far out of line for universal joint absorption. Bad bearing. Loose bellows hose.

Will not tilt or steer: Frozen gimbal ring or gimbal housing bearings. Tilt system out of oil, or dead. Worn zinc trim tab; replace. (See Tilt/Trim.)

Repair Although the stern-drive unit is simple to understand, it is nevertheless heavy and clumsy to handle. Its bearings require special tools for removal and replacement. Stern-drive work often requires shifting of the engine.

The foregoing adds up close to a zero for do-it-yourself repair.

Stoves

A cooking stove has become standard equipment on all pleasure boats with enough enclosed space to house a galley. The choice of fuel varies from alcohol, to kerosene, to some form of gas, to electricity. Cleanest and least troublesome is electricity, although its use means that a generator set must be kept running. Most popular perhaps is alcohol, because its fire may be doused with water. There is also solidified alcohol in cans.

The greatest structural improvements have been made with the electric stove because it has closely followed the household trend. The original spiral elements have been replaced with the solid heating surface, more efficient and easier to clean. Not the least of its attractions is its ability to spruce up the galley after a bit of attention with a damp rag.

The liquid fuel stoves, alcohol and kerosene, operate their burners either by gravity or under pressure. The pressure is obtained with a few strokes of a pump on the stove. A combination electric/alcohol stove also is available and gives skippers the option of running the generator set.

The gas stove, with its infinitely adjustable flame, gives cooks the widest latitude in food preparation. Unfortunately, the thought of explosion always accompanies the word "gas," and the Coast Guard forbids propane on certain passenger-carrying boats. Nevertheless, a correctly installed gas cooking system is eminently safe, especially so when the gas tank is up on deck and protected. Gauges are essential.

The basic factor in determining how to handle a gas is knowing its relationship to air. Is it heavier or lighter than air? Will the fumes fall or rise? This determines what happens with leaks.

STROBE LIGHTS

The lighter gas dissipates in the atmosphere; the heavier gas lodges in the bilge and may become a hazard. The unpleasant odor of a gas is an automatic leak announcer.

The Btu ratings of the fuels provide a comparison of efficacy. One kilowatt of electricity yields 3,400 Btus. One pint of alcohol yields 12,000 Btus. One pound of propane (LPG) yields 21,000 Btus. One pound of natural gas yields 8,000 Btus.

Automatic shut-off of the gas is available. This comes into play if a sudden wind blows out the flame. This is an added safety feature and, of course, adds to the price of the stove.

An ingenious feature on gas stoves is electronic ignition. This is accomplished without recourse to the battery. A piezoelectric material produces a high-voltage spark when compressed.

Electronics is entering the galley to compete with the improved stoves and the modernized fuels. The microwave oven, indispensable for many ashore, is becoming increasingly visible afloat. It is supplied by pier power, by an onboard generating set, or in smaller sizes, by an inverter (see Inverters). Underway, the microwave may interfere with navigational electronics, and even slight aberration of readings can prove serious.

Installation Coast Guard Regulations require gas tanks to be located above decks. Automatic tank shutoffs that work simultaneously with stove shutoffs are desirable. An approved fire extinguisher should be handy to the stove at all times (see Fire Extinguishers).

Maintenance An after-cooking inspection should be made to assure burner shut-off. Burners must be cleaned regularly. Pressure pump gaskets should be checked.

Strobe Lights

The intensely brilliant flashing of a strobe light has proved its lifesaving effectiveness in locating and tracking a man overboard. For this purpose the strobe is fastened to a deck worker's belt or to a life ring kept ready to be thrown. The strobe is activated automatically when it hits the water.

A typical strobe light is built into an orange-colored canister about 12 inches long. The canister holds the battery and the encapsulated solid-state electronic flashing circuit. The light-producing element is a small glass tube filled with xenon gas. A surge of high voltage to the tube excites the gas and produces intense light. (Strobe lights are also available with an incandescent bulb as the light source; the filamentless xenon is preferable.)

In one form of strobe light design, the automatic activation occurs when water reaches the completely dry battery and supplies the moisture an active battery needs. While dry, the battery is inert and has indefinite shelf life.

The canister has a ring for attachment. Various brackets are available for specific needs.

Maintenance A strobe light requires no maintenance other than having it handy and ready—and insisting that it be attached to a deckhand whose work may throw him overboard.

Repair The strobe light is non-repairable.

Stuffing Boxes

The stuffing box makes it possible for the rotating shaft connecting an inboard engine and its propeller to pass through the hull without causing leakage. The device consists of a bronze tube whose inside diameter is much larger than the outside diameter of the shaft. The inboard end of the stuffing box serves to apply axial pressure either with a large gland nut or with an arrangement of studs and nuts. The pressure compacts the greased fibrous material (flax) with which the space between shaft and box is filled.

The filling for the box is available at marine stores in sizes and shapes that may be curled around the shaft. The gland nut, where used, is large in diameter and usually is turned with large-opening so-called water pump pliers. The nuts are within the range of standard wrenches.

Maintenance Maintenance of the stuffing box is controlled by observation: Either there is a leak, meaning that the nuts are too loose (or the filler is worn out), or heat is developed when the shaft is turning, showing that the nuts are too tight. The nuts should be adjusted accordingly.

In the event that proper stuffing box filler cannot be obtained, caulking cotton laced with water pump grease can serve for a short period.

Synchronizers

The twin-engine-boat skipper has the additional problem (though a minor one) of keeping the two engines synchronized in the interest of efficiency and aural comfort. Synchronization means holding the speed of the two power plants to the *exact* same number of revolutions. The exactitude is necessary because each *single* difference in rpm causes an annoying "beat." (A beat sounds somewhat like a tap.)

The human ear is a good synchronizing tool, but it takes a bit of practice. When the engines are started and running at widely different speeds, the beats will be at high frequency and it may be difficult to "pick them out." As the rpm of one engine or the other is changed to match its companion, the beat frequency will decrease and they can be heard distinctly until they cease at perfect synchronism. (The "beat frequency" is simply the difference between the two rpms.)

Perhaps more easily for some skippers, synchronization may also be achieved with electronics. A console light either goes on or goes off at the instant the two engines are running exactly even. Some synchronizers or "syncs" are combined with tachometers because they depend on the same ignition pulses from the engines. (The need for ignition pulses restricts the use of this type of synchronizer and ta-

TACHOMETERS

chometer to gasoline engine. Some form of pulse generator must be added for diesels.)

Active synchronizers are available that hold the engines to synchronous running without manual aid. Naturally, these are complicated mechanisms far removed from the mere indicators. They may be obtained for both gas and diesel engines. An added bonus from these mechanical synchronizers is that both engines may be controlled simultaneously with one throttle level.

Installation The continuous stream of electrical pulses to the synchronizer may be "annoying" to other console instruments. Careful placement is required. Capacitors may need to be added (see Static).

Tachometers

A tachometer measures the speed of rotation—on a boat, the rpm of the engine. A "tach" may achieve its readings in several ways, depending upon its internal design: It may function as a frequency meter calibrated in rpm (revolutions per minute), or it may be a voltmeter with rpm calibration. The form of action is mated to the kind of sender attached to the engine.

Installation Gasoline engines allow the easiest tachometer additions because the rate of interruption of the ignition current bears a direct ratio to rpm. The tachometer simply measures the frequency of the ignition current breaks and adjusts for two- or four-cycle and number of cylinders. Thus, a two-wire connection from tach to engine does the trick.

With a diesel engine, the installation becomes more complicated because ignition current is absent. One method installs a breaker-point device at the engine's tachometer outlet; the frequency of breaks then is read by the tachometer, as with the gasoline engine. Another scheme installs a small direct-current generator at this same outlet in place of the breaker. The voltage output of this generator is exactly proportionate to rpm, allowing a simple voltmeter to be calibrated in engine speed. In both cases, a two-wire conductor between engine and tach suffices.

The market offers a choice between the analog readouts of a pointer on a meter scale and a digital readout on a screen. The numerals are formed by liquid crystals and are clear even in sunlight. The breaks from the engine are transformed into numerals by a solid-state electronic circuit within the display housing.

Maintenance The accuracy of the readouts may be checked with a manual rpm counter and a stopwatch. (A stroboscopic counter "reads" a mark on the flywheel. The strobe speed is varied until the mark appears to stand still.)

Thermostats

A thermostat is a control device that performs a desired function at a preset temperature. Thermostats monitor engine coolant temperature, refrigerator temperature, and the desired comfort level of airconditioning.

A thermostat is built to conform to one of three styles of internal construction of its actuating element. For engine coolant monitoring (see Engines), this element is a sealed bellows. For refrigeration, the element is a sealed, gas-filled sensor connected to the thermostat by a metal tube (see Refrigeration). The element in the airconditioning thermostat is a calibrated, bimetallic spring (see Airconditioning).

The bellows of the coolant thermostat may contain a gas for more accurate and stronger reaction. The expansion of the bellows moves a damper valve that restricts coolant flow. At the designed temperature, the valve opens and relinquishes control. Thermostats of this type are not adjustable and are selected for a desired temperature.

The sensor in the refrigerator thermostat responds to the temperature in the cooling system and opens and closes a switch in the driving motor circuit. This thermostat is calibrated in degrees and is adjustable by the user.

The airconditioning thermostat monitors the temperature of the air being delivered to the conditioned space. It, too, "makes and breaks" a switch in the motor circuit in order to maintain a set point. The set point is adjustable over a wide range.

Maintenance The calibration of an engine thermostats may be checked easily. The thermostat is placed in a pan of water on a stove, together with a thermometer. The water is heated gradually while the thermometer is watched. The valve should open at a temperature close to that specified for the thermostat.

Verifying the calibration of the refrigerator thermostat is done with a reliable thermometer that is known to be accurate in the 40-degree area (the probable set point of the refrigerator).

The accuracy of the airconditioning thermostat calibration may be checked only indirectly. After verifying room temperature, the thermostat adjustment is moved slowly until the switch click is heard. The temperature reading at the click should be identical with room temperature.

Repair Replacing an engine thermostat is not difficult. Thermostats usually are located at or near the point where hot coolant leaves the engine; the exact location is given in the owner's manual, together with the steps necessary for removal.

A defective engine thermostat is not repairable.

Tides and Currents

Skippers who cruise the coastal waters and their connecting rivers are affected by two additional facets of Nature with which they should be familiar: tides and currents. These two water movements are often mistakenly considered analogous; they are *not*. Tides cause the rise and fall in the height of the water. Currents move water from one place to another. Nevertheless, tides and currents are interdependent, with the former often the cause of the latter.

Tides result from the forces exerted on the waters of the Earth's oceans by celestial bodies. The sun and the moon

TIDES AND CURRENTS

wield gravitational force proportional to their size, positions, and distance from Earth. The Earth adds to its gravitational power the centrifugal power caused by celestial rotation. Nature combines these various forces into a changing but repetitive pattern that makes it possible for tides and currents to be predicted for the mariner. The predictions are based on government-calculated tables.

Each month, when the moon is full and again when the moon is new, the forces line up and add to each other to have the greatest effect on tides. Such tides are at maximum and are called "spring" tides (a name, not a season). In between, at first-quarter moon and at third-quarter moon, the forces are at right angles and not fully additive, and the effect on tides is minimal. Such tides are called "neap" tides.

The moon is the closest of the celestial bodies that govern tides, and therefore it is the major contributor to the tidal forces. However, the moon varies in its distance from Earth, and this varies the intensity of its effects. The effect, and the consequent tidal range, are greatest when the moon is closest, at perigee, and are least when the moon is farthest, at apogee. The moon condition lags by 50 minutes each day because the moon takes 50 minutes more than 24 hours to encircle the Earth.

The effects of tide are not universally identical at all points on tidal waters. When there are two approximately even high tides and two approximately equal lows, occurring within 24 hours, the condition is known as "semidiurnal." One high and one low in 24 hours would make them "diurnal" tides. When the high and low ranges are unequal, it becomes a "mixed" tide. Generally speaking, the semidiurnal tides are found on the East Coast and the mixed tides on the West Coast. The cause of these variations is geophysical.

The critical tide question of a cruising skipper is whether or not there is sufficient water to float his vessel safely, regardless of tide. Often the answer may be had directly from the chart, because charted depths are based on "mean low water." When this depth alone is insufficient, then resort to tidal tables becomes necessary.

The National Ocean Service (NOS) is the disseminator of tidal information in the form of tide tables, and these are available where charts are sold. The tables take the form of "reference stations" and "subordinate stations" and, between them, cover all locations of boating interest. All publications are revised yearly; outdated tables should not be used.

The method of recovering tidal information is first to consult the nearest reference-station table for the basic data. The subordinate-station table containing the location of interest is then used to obtain the corrections for time and height. In addition, tidal ranges are given for neap and spring tides. An additional table permits the calculation of actual tidal height at any selected time between low and high.

Water seeks a common level, and when tidal effects cause a difference in height of water at two points, a flow, a "tidal current," will take place. Currents are numerous in the oceans of the Earth where they are virtually "rivers in the sea"; among the causes are wind, the forces generated by the Earth's rotation, by the shapes of the continents. Rivers have currents due to tides and to the natural function of drainage.

A current is described by its "set" and by its "drift." The set of a current is the geographic direction in which it flows. The drift of a current is the speed of the flow in knots or miles per hour. A tidal current coming in from the ocean is at "flood," and when returning it is at "ebb." The time of reversal of a tidal current is a period of no water flow, called "slack water." The tidal term "stand" represents a condition wherein the height of tide at a certain point does not change, even though some flow of water continues.

Currents can have a direct effect on the course and speed of a vessel afloat in them (see Wind/Current vs. Course). When the set and the course are the same, conditions are additive; set and course agree, drift adds to boat speed. At all other angles, the results are vectorial. The skipper of a slow boat must be very watchful of his arithmetic and of his steering.

Tidal current predictions follow much the same route as those for the tides, and this, too, is a service of the National Ocean Services (NOS). As with tides, there are "reference stations," lists of subordinate stations, and intermediate flow tables. Current flow diagrams are supplied for important coastal points. Additional current details are available from NOS in the form of charts of important coastal locations with the pertinent currents identified by arrows. The effects of current on the speed and course of a boat are solved best by plotting vectorially.

Course and set are laid down as lines at angles. Speed and drift determine the lengths of these lines in suitably chosen units. The closure of the triangles carries the solutions. (See Plotting and Vectors.)

Tilt/Trim

Both outboard motors and stern-drive units have the ability to swing up and down, and thereby regulate the angle of attack of the propeller against the water. Thus, the most efficient angle may be chosen to suit the local conditions of load, speed, hull design, or whatever.

Early models of outboards had only a pin and a series of holes with which to fix the tilt position. The pin was placed in a selected hole, and it set the tilt by resting against a stop. The operator was restricted to four or five holes and an equivalent number of positions. Obviously, the modification in tilt could not be made underway, as the unit had to be stopped.

Modern tilt installations are totally opposite. Tilt changes may be made while at speed, and any angle between the up and the down limits may be chosen. The only effort involved in doing this is to push the tilt buttons on the console. The work is performed by a hydraulic system.

The system has variations when applied to various models of outboards and stern-drives, but the essentials are the same. Oil, either under low or high pressure, forces rods back and forth in

TILT/TRIM

control cylinders; this lifts or drops the outboard or stern-drive in the selected direction and holds it there. The pressure and movement are under the command of the console push buttons.

The oil pressure is generated by an electric motor-driven pump running on battery voltage. A safety switch or valve prevents the motor from being actuated when the gear shift is in reverse. (The forces would be in ruinous opposition.) An extra button on the control console raises the outboard or stern-drive to the extra height required for safe trailering. All tilt movements are sensed by a sender and reported to the console, where they are displayed on a trim gauge. A trim angle in which the cavitation plate is horizontal is considered neutral for most boats.

The cavitation plate is the flat surface directly over the propeller and is found in all stern-drives and outboards except the very smallest (see Cavitation). This plate also carries the trim tab, a small rudder-like vane that balances out the undesirable sideward thrust of a propeller (see Trim Tabs). The trim tab does double duty by being made of zinc and acting as a protective anode (see Electrolysis).

Maintenance Maintenance for tilt/trim units boils down to lubrication, maintenance of oil pump reservoir levels, and visual inspection to verify that the hoses are properly dressed and cannot kink. A few runs of the unit from limit to limit should verify the inspection.

The oil for the pump of the low-pressure models is *not* the same as the correct oil for the high-pressure units. The owner's manual identifies the right oil for each, and separates the high-pressure from the low-pressure designs. One manufacturer specifies regular automotive oil for the high-pressure hydraulic systems and auto transmission fluid for the low-pressure systems. The usual instructions are to fill the reservoir to a level even with filler or inspection hole. Overfilling (by closing the hole) can damage the electric-motor pump drive.

Oil contamination is generally at the root of electric motor failure and must be guarded against. One cause is a failing pump shaft seal; another is overloading through malfunction; still another is entry of moisture. Applying a thin coat of waterproof gook to all suspected areas of the motor housing is worthwhile.

Troubleshooting Tilt/trim troubleshooting logic: this is an electromechanical device, so malfunction must be either electrical or mechanical (hydraulic) but rarely both. The mechanical members are exposed for visual inspection. The electrical portion includes console buttons, limit switches, an electric motor, and wiring from battery to unit. In addition, sensors connect to console gauges and continuously show the boat operator the exact position of the tilt/trim unit. Visual comparison, of what the gauges are reporting and what exactly is taking place, checks the sensor system.

Button pushed, pump does not run: Low battery. Open circuit. Gear in reverse. Overload (excess temperature) switch in motor open. Burned-out motor. Hydraulic (excess pressure) lockup.

Responds to either up or down button but not to both: One wire off. Defective button. Defective solenoid. Low fluid level. Ground off or corroded. Reverse cut-out safety switch stuck.

Erratic movement of tilt/trim: Low fluid level. Trapped air in system.

Unit rises but will not go high enough for safe trailering: Middle button defective. Wire off middle button. Upper limit switch defective.

Current draw test: (This test should be made with an "induction" ammeter that requires no cutting or disconnecting of wires.) Raising the tilt/trim requires approximately twice the power for lowering, and the up ampere reading should be approximately twice the down amperes. (See Volt and Ampere Meters.)

Repair A common problem with a tilt/trim that has seen long service is failure to hold its set position underway. This indicates check valve leakage and becomes a professional repair. The replacement of hydraulic hoses is within the boatman's purview if carefully performed according to the instructions in the owner's manual.

Transducers

A transducer is a device that accepts energy in one form and delivers it in another form. The most common form of transducer aboard is probably the one connected to the depthsounder and projecting downward through the hull. It accepts energy in the form of high-frequency alternating current from the sounder and transforms it into a sonic beam that reflects from the bottom and from fish. The transducer changes the reflection back into an alternating current that becomes the sounder reading.

Transducer construction may be piezoelectric or electromagnetic. (Piezo

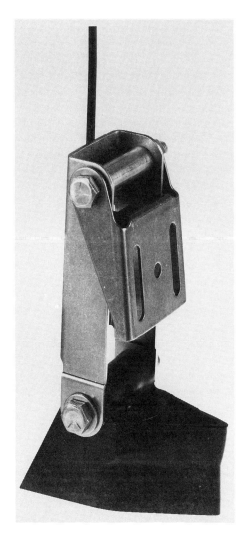

TRANSDUCERS—This modern transducer for a depthsounder is shown complete with an adjustable transom-attachment bracket. *(Courtesy Lowrance Electronics)*

elements are minerals that generate electrical currents when they are flexed.) The operating element in the piezo style is a crystal (quartz or synthetic) that emits an electric current when stressed. The electromechanical style contains a magnetic winding upon a ferrous core. In the transducer's "send" pattern, electric current from the sounder stresses the crystal or the winding and forms and projects the sonic beam. The reverse action from a reflected sound generates the answering current for the sounder display.

Transducers may cover a wide band of frequencies or, as in depthsounder work, they may be tuned to a narrow resonance, such as 50 kilohertz or 200 kilohertz. (The lower frequency is for deep sounding.) The housing for run-of-the-mill transducers is plastic, but higher-grade units are manufactured with bronze. The housing has a threaded neck that projects through the hull, contains the connecting cable, and fastens with a nut.

Installation The most popular positioning of transducers for depthsounders is amidships, through the hull, and far enough away from a projecting keel to prevent obstructing the sonic beam. The axis of the transducer must be vertical with the ship in correct trim. The transducer must remain fully immersed regardless of trim.

It is possible, by various methods, to keep the transducer inside the hull and avoid holing. This convenience is had at the cost of sensitivity, but many sounders have sufficient power to overcome the drawback (see Depthsounders).

Since most hull bottoms have roundness, the vertical position of the transducer is attained by shaped filler pieces between hull and transducer housing.

Installation of a transducer in the hull generally requires hauling out. However, there is a trick that allows transducer installation while afloat. A long wooden stick is made ready with a strong fish line attached to one end. The hole is drilled, the stick is pushed forcefully through, and the hole is plugged with rags. The stick is retrieved, and the transducer is given the fish line. The transducer is hauled in through the hole. (A flamboyant job! It's been done, but it is not recommended.)

Maintenance Maintenance for transducers consists in keeping them clean and free of marine growths. This should be mandatory at every hauling. Transducers should not be painted. An advantage of the transom–mount for transducers is the ease of service (see Hauling Out).

Troubleshooting The only non-laboratory check of the effectiveness of a transducer is to substitute a known good unit for the questionable one and compare results.

Repair Transducers are not repairable. They should be kept clear of fouling by gentle scrubbing with bronze wool.

Transformers

An electric transformer may be as small as a pea and functioning as a unit of an electronic circuit, or it may be the monster in the field of the power sta-

TRANSMISSIONS

tion. In both cases, the purpose of the transformer is the same: to transfer energy from one circuit to another, while keeping the circuits isolated from each other.

A transformer consists of two windings upon a core. The two windings are called "primary" and "secondary." The relationship of primary and secondary voltages is determined by the ratio of the number of turns of wire in these two windings. For electronic work, the core may be powdered iron or air. For service at commercial frequencies, the core is always built up of layers of iron sheets.

The transformer most likely to come within the ken of the skipper forms a part of the battery charger. Here it isolates the battery from the pier and reduces the commercial 120 volts to the 12 volts of the battery.

Repair Under certain deleterious conditions, transformers are subject to flashover and burnout. When this happens, they are non-repairable and must be replaced. Transformers are classified by voltage and power-handling capacity.

Transistors

All modern marine electronic equipment depends upon transistors for its functioning. Transistors are also known as "semiconductors." The transistor is "solid state," so-called because it consists of a sandwich of two rare doped minerals; it has no moving parts. ("Doping," in the semiconductor industry, signifies adding a minute amount of a foreign chemical to a crystal.) Electrons carry the desired current of a circuit in a manner predetermined, by design, to achieve a certain result, be it communication or direction finding or radar or whatever. The small bulk of transistors has made possible the remarkable miniaturization of all electronic devices.

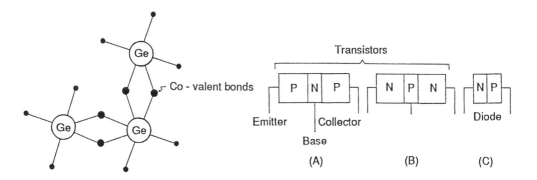

TRANSISTORS—The drawings show how the doped germanium material is bonded together, atom to atom. The transistor is a "sandwich" as shown. The diode is half a transistor. N and P germanium are the results of two styles of dopings. ("Doping" is the introduction of minute amounts of foreign matter.)

TRANSMISSIONS

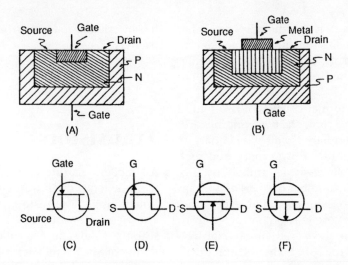

TRANSISTORS—Two improvements in transistors are shown here in cross-sectional construction. At (A) is the field effect transistor, at (B) the Mosfet (metal oxide field effect) transistor. Both exhibit greater sensitivity and less noise. The symbols portraying the various modes of connection are shown.

Hordes of transistor types are available on the market, each one with specifications that make it the choice for a given job. The most important specs are voltage and current-carrying ability. Mini power transistors are pea-size and are soldered onto circuit boards by their leads (see Soldering). Large power transistors are mounted on "heat sinks" to dissipate what otherwise would be destructive heat (see Heat Sinks).

Transistors are not degraded by usage; they don't wear out when in a properly designed circuit and, theoretically, could last "forever."

Troubleshooting Heat, and the overloading that causes heat, are the death-dealing enemies of transistors. A common mistake is to "key" a transmitter without having the antenna attached. The antenna-less, unbalanced circuit quickly overloads and overheats the radio power transistor and destroys it.

Transmissions

Internal-combustion engines cannot be sequentially started and stopped and must run continuously during their working period. The starting, stopping, and reversing are performed by a device called a "transmission" placed between the engine and the propeller shaft. The internal functioning of this transmission may be manual or hydraulic. Usually also, the transmission includes gearing whose ratio matches the engine characteristics to the propeller load.

The manual transmission is oper-

TRANSMISSIONS

ated by an attached lever. The hydraulic transmission is under the control of an internal high-pressure oil system that responds to a remote cable. A safety switch permits the engine to start only when the transmission is in "neutral," meaning that no engine rotation is being transmitted.

A common design of transmissions uses a friction clutch to couple the engine to the propeller for forward motion. The lever of the manual unit and the oil-pressured piston of the hydraulic unit each activate this clutch. For reverse, a brake band is activated to hold the outer case of a planetary gear to cause a reversal of the output rotation of the engine. (A "planetary" system has gears within gears, and its movement duplicates the action of the sun and its planets.) Rotation is labeled "right" or "left" (clockwise or counterclockwise) as seen by looking at the output end of the engine or transmission.

An efficient engine speed is usually higher than an efficient propeller speed. The optimum match between the two is accomplished by the reduction gearing in the transmission,

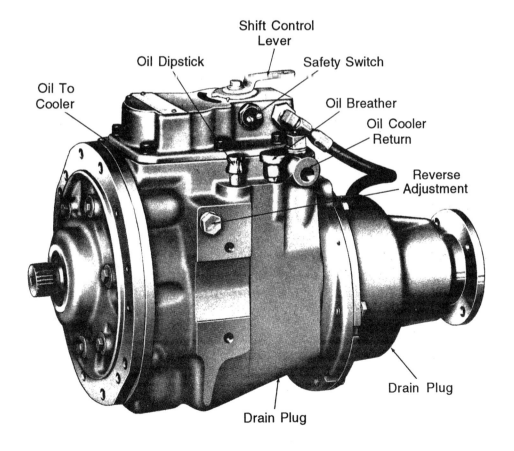

TRANSMISSIONS

wherein a smaller gear drives a larger gear. Some popular gear ratios are 1½ to 1, 2 to 1, even 3 to 1.

A boat engine is always pushing "up a hill," never coasting like an automobile. This puts marine transmission gearing under constant stress and requires cooling. The hydraulic transmission fluid (the same as used in automobile automatic transmissions) is cooled by passage through a heat exchanger. Lubrication is either shared with the engine, or it is entirely independent.

Installation In a standard installation, the transmission housing is bolted to the engine. Power is transmitted from the engine to the transmission via a splined hole and a matching splined shaft. Concentricity is assured by the bolted housing. A flange at the output of the transmission accepts the flange on the propeller shaft. Concentricity here is essential to avoid vibration, noise, and wear; the perfect line-up is achieved by trial and error, using a .002-inch shim as a gauge.

Engine, transmission, and shaft are moved, a hair this way, a hair that, until the trial shim between the flanges is held with equal tightness all around. Only when this condition is reached should the shim be removed and the flanges be bolted together. Final tightening of all mounting bolts follows.

Maintenance Independently lubricated modern marine transmissions require only the simplest, commonsense maintenance, and this consists essentially of maintaining oil quantity and quality. While this sounds easy enough, the actual performance of this maintenance may be messy because of the transmission's location.

The gist of the instructions is to routinely check the dipstick to ensure that there is sufficient oil, and to change the oil at the specified intervals. The owner's manual is the bible on frequency of oil changes. One popular manufacturer wants the transmission oil changed "every 100 hours of each season under normal use." Only the specific type and viscosity of oil called for in the owner's manual should be used. Any filters in the system will need to be replaced when oil is changed. It is wise to run the engine a few minutes after an oil change and then to recheck the dipstick to ensure that all passages are filled.

The dipstick is the gauge that determines quantity. A caution here is to make sure the dipstick is correct for the transmission. (Misplaced dipsticks are not that unusual.)

Visual inspection for oil leaks is a good habit to acquire. The transmission housing should be kept clean so that leaks may quickly be detected. Part of your inspection should be to compare the position of the remote shift lever and the shift lever on the transmission, to verify that they agree. The safety switch that permits engine starting only in neutral should be tested. (See Engines.)

Troubleshooting Troubleshooting a transmission is made easier because whatever could be at fault is located within a small, exposed housing. Logical analysis starts with an engine running correctly and feeding power into the front end of the transmission. Is that power being handled in accordance with the request of the gear-shift level? For instance, with the shift in neutral, is the propeller shaft turning

TRIM TABS

nevertheless? Or is the shaft motionless despite the shift lever being in reverse? (Solutions differ for manual and for hydraulaic units.)

Shift in neutral, prop shaft turns: Dragging forward, clutch adjustment too tight. Dragging reverse, planetary band too tight.

Shift in forward or reverse, prop shaft stopped: Check clutch adjustment for forward, band adjustment for reverse. (Also if prop shaft is sluggish.) On hydraulic units, check internal oil supply. Worst case: Catastrophic failure of clutch plates or gear train.

Slippage under load, shift forward or reverse: Worn clutch plates. Reverse band worn. Low oil in hydraulic unit.

Oil leaks on housing: Oil over fuel mark on dipstick. Worn or damaged gaskets and seals. Overheated unit and excreting from breather.

Repair As stated above, the trouble is easier to find because it is all within one housing. Unfortunately, that does not make it easier to fix. Making slight adjustments in clutch operations, as above, is as far as the do-it-yourself skipper can go with a modern transmission. Repairing transmissions is a messy job that requires experience with gearing and close tolerances. The skipper had best leave the work to a professional shop.

Trim Tabs

Small boats are unduly responsive in their trim to the weight and position of the load carried aboard. Unless weight is minimal and position ideal, the boat will "squat" and use its power inefficiently. A common antidote is the use of trim tabs, adjustable flat surfaces extending from the lower edge of the stern and controlled from the console.

Trim tabs use the hydraulic reaction of the water passing under the stern to push the stern up, the bow down, and thereby to correct trim. The force needed to hold the trim tabs in position is supplied by hydraulic pressure from a battery-operated pump. Joystick or pushbutton controls regulate the pressure to maintain the proper balance of forces.

Ordinarily, the trim of outboard and stern-drive boats is altered by changing the angle of propeller thrust. This is inefficient because the ideal direction of thrust is parallel with the surface of the water. At any other angle, a portion of engine power is subtracted from forward drive and used for trimming. Adding trim tabs leaves the engine free to push the boat as its only job. The correction of squatting puts less load on the engine for a given speed.

Installation The optimum size of trim tabs is governed by the size, speed, type, and displacement of the boat, and manufacturers publish tables of recommendations. For instance, a 16-foot runabout is fitted with trim tabs less than 1 square foot in area, while a 70-foot vessel needs trim tabs that measure 6 square feet. The trim tab assembly is screwed to the transom according to instructions and is supplied through the transom by hydraulic tubing.

A final touch to the installation is the addition of indicators to the con-

TROUBLE LAMPS

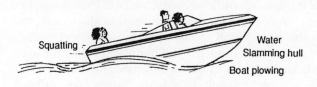
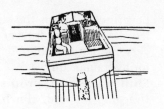

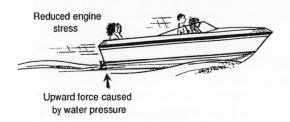
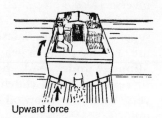

TRIM TABS—Trim tabs transform a very small fraction of the boat's thrust into a trimming force to be applied when needed. *(Courtesy Bennett)*

sole that show the exact position of the trim tabs. Knowledge of this nature is especially helpful when the trim tabs are suppoed to be fully retracted. Sensors at the trim tabs (in the cylinders) pick up the information and sent it forward electrically.

Maintenance The trim tab hydraulic system is filled with automobile automatic transmission fluid. Occasional inspection should be made to verify the level.

A zinc anode should be screwed to each trim tab for boats in salt water. When used in locations subject to heavy fouling, the trim tabs should be wirebrushed and painted with a recommended antifouling paint according to the directions on the can.

The fuse protecting the hydraulic pump should be cut into the "hot" wire no more than 6 feet from the battery; this is a Coast Guard regulation.

Trouble Lamps

Two easily assembled light bulb units are unmatched for troubleshooting electrical circuits. One is useful on all battery voltage circuits that are giving trouble. The other is used on both 120-volt and 240-volt circuits.

The low-voltage tester consists of a low-candlepower 12-volt bulb, such as an automobile license plate light. An 8-inch piece of flexible wire with one

TROUBLE LAMPS

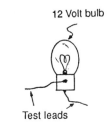

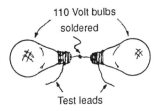

TROUBLE LAMPS—These quickly assembled trouble lamps will prove a blessing when circuits must be checked. The small bulb tests all the low-voltage wiring on the boat. The double bulb is used on 120-volt and 240-volt circuits—bright on 240, dim on 120.

end bared is soldered to the base contact; a similar wire is soldered to the base shell (see Soldering). That's all there is to it; its usefulness far exceeds its simplicity.

The high-voltage tester requires two 120-volt bulbs of the type known as night lights and rated 7 watts. The two bulbs are united by soldering their base contacts together as shown. An 8-inch piece of flexible wire with one end bared is then soldered to each base shell. The combined base section is then insulated *thoroughly* with electrical tape. Better still, the entire base area may be encased in any hard-setting resin compound.

The high-voltage tester may be used on any 120-volt or 240-volt circuit. It automatically identifies the voltage: The bulbs will be dim on 120 and bright on 240.

The various troubleshooting procedures make use of the lights to ascertain whether or not voltage is present at a point of doubt. They draw too little current to upset any circuit.

TROUBLE CHART

ACTION	QUESTION	ANSWER	SEE
TURN INSTRUMENT ON	DOES PILOT LIGHT?	YES NO	1 2
CONNECT TROUBLE LAMP TO INSTRUMENT TERMINALS	DOES TROUBLE LAMP LIGHT?	YES NO	3 4
CHECK FUSE	CONTINUITY?	YES NO	5 6
CHECK BATTERY	SPECIFIC GRAVITY?	AROUND 1200 MUCH LOWER	7 8
CHECK SWITCH	CONTACT?	GOOD NO	9 10

TV Afloat

The dependence on television that the public has developed makes it natural to expect many TV receivers to be installed on pleasure boats. But the quality of TV reception afloat is below that considered optimum ashore. The reason is twofold: restricted antenna size and insufficient antenna height.

The market offers several designs of TV antennas for boats. Active and passive styles are available. The active antennas contain boosting amplifiers while the passive units are merely antennas. Power for the active amplifiers is sent up on the downlead.

Some antennas are rotatable from a remote control at the receiver; this takes advantage of the directional character of antennas to draw the maximum energy from the passing wave. Placing the boosting amplifier directly into the antenna allows the TV signal to be strengthened before it arrives in areas that produce electrical noise contamination.

Shapewise, marine TV antennas vary. Some are contained in round, flat pielike housings. Others are a central unit with two extending arms. Some boats make do with "rabbit ears."

Maintenance TV antennas require no maintenance other than being wiped free of salt spray.

Universal Joints

Often a local condition makes it impossible to keep the input and the output of a shaft in the same straight line. Such a problem may be solved with universal joints.

A universal joint consists of a short shaft connecting two gimbal-like devices, each of which is free to swing a full 360 degrees. Turning one end turns the other, even when the two ends are out of line. However, the turns will not coincide, degree by degree, unless the universal joint is designed as a "constant-velocity unit." (The advent of front-wheel-drive automobiles has brought a large demand for this type of universal joint.)

Aboard a boat, universal joints may be found in the propulsion power line (see Stern-Drives), in the steering system, and perhaps for special applications.

Maintenance Universal joints require adequate lubrication and protection from dirt. This latter requirement may be met with a covering "boot," a leather enclosure.

Vapor Alarms

Considering the amount of explosive cargo in the form of gasoline carried by a powerboat, it is amazing how rarely one hears of a fire aboard. The reasons for the record of safety are the careful handling that becomes habitual for the skipper, the wide use of vapor alarms, and—not least, by any means—the human nose.

The nose is an extremely sensitive detector of flammable fumes. A sniff of the bilge before starting the engine(s) comprises free insurance against disaster, and should also signal the turning

VAPOR ALARMS

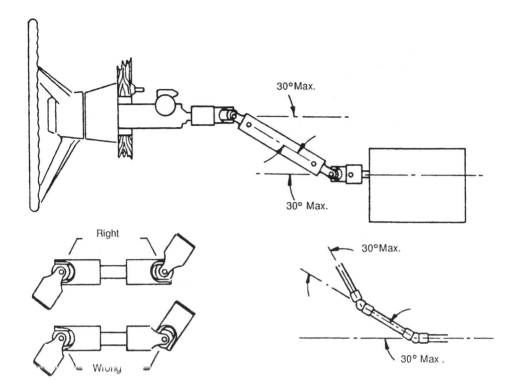

UNIVERSAL JOINTS—The use of a universal joint in the steering system is shown. Note the special instruction about the correct mechanical relationship of the two ends. *(Courtesy Benmar)*

on of the bilge blowers (see Bilge Blowers).

Vapor alarms are available in wide variety. The better models do not restrict their sniffing to the fumes of gasoline but also detect cooking gases like propane, LPG (liquid petroleum gas), and LNG (liquified natural gas), all of which are heavier than air and gather low in the bilge. One vapor alarm is responsive to carbon monoxide; it is intended for gasoline-powered cabin boats with long exhaust pipes that may come under suspicion.

One method of operation of vapor alarms depends upon a platinum wire. The wire is kept at constant temperature by means of a carefully regulated electric current. A flammable vapor "burns" on the wire and raises its temperature. This upsets the circuit and energizes the alarms.

The standard vapor alarms announce the presence of danger by activating red lights and horns.

Most alarms have a button with which the bilge condition may be tested before starting the engine.

Troubleshooting Routine testing of the vapor alarm (in addition to the self-test) may be done by bringing a rag spinkled with a few drops of gasoline near the sensor.

Repair Sensors may go bad for

VARIABLE-RATIO OILING (VRO)

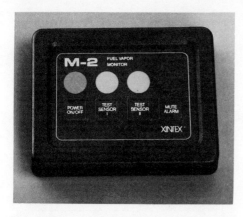

VAPOR ALARMS—When the vapor alarm is turned on, it sniffs the bilge continuously for dangerous fumes. (Its rival is the human nose.) *(Courtesy Xintex)*

many reasons, not all preventable. Manufacturers all supply extra sensors at proportionate cost; installation entails a simple cable connection.

Variable-Ratio Oiling (VRO)

Two-stroke-cycle outboard motors use the crankcase as part of the fuel system and consequently have no place for an oil lamp. The oil must be added to the gasoline, and it is burned as part of the charge.

Oil and gasoline must bear a fixed ratio (given in the owner's manual). Originally this ratio was as small as 10 to 1; naturally, it caused smoke in the exhaust. Improved formulations for lubricating oil permit the ratio to be raised considerably for today's engines. A representative ratio now is 50 to 1 and, with special oils, even 100 to 1.

Obviously, this careful mixing is a chore, and a new development has come forth to eliminate it: variable-ratio oiling (VRO).

VRO is accomplished by a special oil pump that is an inherent part of the fuel pump. This pump operates on engine vacuum and uses the degree of vacuum to gauge the engine load and the resulting need for more or less oil to be squirted into the fuel. The resulting ratio may vary from 25 to 1, to 150 to 1. The oil is taken from a small tank.

The makers of VRO suggest careful observation to make certain the oil is actually being pumped. They suggest a safety measure: At startup, oil should also be mixed with the fuel at a ratio of 50 to 1, to give the VRO time to catch up.

Maintenance Maintenance for the VRO unit consists in keeping all hoses tight to exclude the entry of air that would "kill" system operation by obscuring engine vacuum.

Troubleshooting Troubleshooting logic: The VRO needs vacuum and available oil. Check hoses for tightness and obstruction. Check the oil tank level. A screwdriver "stethoscope" should make workings in the pump audible (see Engines).

Varnishes

In days not too long gone, the pleasure-boating scene owed much of its

VARNISHES

eye appeal to beautifully varnished surfaces. That attraction is now seen less frequently, together with the wooden vessels that featured it. Varnish no longer is a commonly used protective coating—although the material itself has lost none of its effectiveness and, in fact, has been improved. The old-time straight varnish has been moved relatively into the background by the many new clear synthetics that give better results and longer service.

Ancient boatbuilders used a protective coating that could be considered a primitive varnish. They diluted a resin from trees with oil. This fluid was allowed to soak deeply into the wood to protect against the environment and the prevalent bugs.

Modern varnish generally chooses from five ingredients whose proportions may vary greatly with different manufacturers. The oil of choice today is tung oil, also known as China wood oil, derived from trees. The resin is synthetic. Added also are solvents, driers, and specialized chemicals to prevent premature skinning of the surface. The sun is the greatest enemy of varnish, and so all exterior varnishes contain a chemical to neutralize the effects of ultraviolet rays. Most varnish applications dry overnight. The trade rates varnish as "long" or "short," depending upon the percentage of oil in the formula.

Applying varnish is 90 percent preparation and 10 percent application. The major portion of preparation is devoted to sanding, with filling and bleaching added when necessary. The sandpaper chosen for the beginning is generally around 80 grit, with progressively higher numbers as the surface improves. Light sanding after each coat has the goal of a flat, smooth surface. A filler (if the surface requires it) is brushed across the grain and wiped level before it dries hard.

The difference in working with paint and with varnish lies in the technique of application. Paint is brushed on and brushed out to a thin coat. Varnish is "flowed" on, with no back-and-forth brush strokes for leveling. Varnish does not have the "body" of paint and requires many more coats than paint. The ideal environment for varnishing includes the absence of sun, no wind, low humidity, and temperature around 70 degrees Fahrenheit. The day's varnishing should end early enough to permit surface drying before dew sets in.

It is customary to run a can of paint through a shaking machine before use to stir up the ingredients that have separated by gravity. This should *not* be done with varnish, because it would introduce air bubbles that interfere with smooth application. Experts move the varnish can as little as possible; they pour off a small amount for immediate use and avoid dipping the brush into the varnish can, which causes bubbles. (A brush only partially loaded with varnish also can cause air bubbles.)

Chilling the varnish in a refrigerator for use on a hot day may be worth a try. This could help in blending brush strokes.

If old varnish must be removed, three methods are available: sandpaper, chemicals, and heat. Sandpapering is a good, all-around method, but a thick coat of varnish can make it self-

VECTORS

defeating because of the clogging and smudging of the paper. Power sanders save time and effort. Chemical removers can lift the old coat of varnish so that it may be removed with a putty knife. (Some chemical removers require neutralizing.) Heat from a blow torch or heat gun brings the danger of damaging the wood. Heat must be applied carefully and removed the instant the paint softens and swells (amateurs often leave the heat on too long).

Vectors

A vector is a line of proportionate given length, drawn in a given direction. A vector by its length and angle, may represent any condition of direction and velocity, as, for instance, the direction (set) of a current and its velocity (drift). Vectors make it possible to solve geometric problems graphically, without recourse to numerical calculations. The necessary tools are only pencil, paper, protractor, and scale.

The ideal condition of boat movement occurs when the dead reckoning (DR) track and the course made good over the bottom are identical; this takes place only when current and wind are both absent. When wind and/or current are affecting progress, the amount of help or hindrance may quickly be reduced to workable numbers by using vectors. (The combined effect of wind and current and other factors may be handled as one vector.)

The vector solution may specify the necessary steering correction to cross to a point directly opposite on a river with current (see Plotting). A vector can predict the difference between the intended course and speed and the actual "course over the ground" (COG) and "speed over the ground" (SOG) caused by local conditions. In all cases, the solution involves vector triangles in which two sides are given and the third side, the answer, is merely the vector needed to complete the enclosure.

A logical explanation will help clear the mind on the effects of current. Assume travel due north at 10 knots. Assume a current of 2 knots flowing to the east. It is obvious that for every 10 miles the boat goes north, it will also go 2 miles east. Connecting this final position with the origin results in a vector statement of what took place.

It is customary to label all vectors, above the line for course and below the line for speed. Vector calculations may be drawn directly on the chart but preferably are made on separate sheets of paper.

Ventilation Systems

Common sense and the Coast Guard both require that enclosed spaces occupied by gasoline engines or gasoline tanks be properly ventilated. Natural, gravity ventilation alone is not sufficient and not legal. The air must be moved by a powered blower through ducts of mandated minimum cross section (see Bilge Blowers).

Installation In almost all installations, the blower motor is a direct-current type run by the storage battery. Such a motor has a commutator and brushes and may be a source of dangerous sparks. Consequently, this motor may not be placed low in the bilge. It should be located as high in the vented area as possible and suck out vapors through a suction duct from the lowest dry point in the bilge.

Coast Guard regulations require the presence of natural, gravity ventilation ducts in addition to the forced air. Although an escape clause permits nonconformance with the regulations upon proof of certain "open" constructions, it is advisable to provide all the ventilation possible nevertheless. All present builders of boats provide means for excess ventilation, and older boats should be brought to the same level of safety.

The passive portion of the ventilation system is designed to take its air movement from the ram effect of the forward travel of the boat. An extended cowl at the intake exerts pressure, and a cowl at the discharge creates vacuum. The two outside cowls mark the extent of the engine or tank compartment. The duct from the intake cowl must reach down at least to below carburetor level. The output duct must be in the bilge but high enough to avoid being blocked by bilgewater.

Although the rules require only one two-cowl system per engine, builders supply one to port and one to starboard, even on single-engine boats. Builders are required to prove the air-handling capability of the exhaust systems, but this is rarely expected of an owner-skipper.

The ventilation system must not overlook or interfere with the carburetor's need for large quantities of air for internal combustion. This air is brought into the engine compartment through spray-protected openings. Diesels are massive gulpers of air.

To assure correct use of the blower, the blower switch should be located at the ignition switch with a small instruction panel. The instructions state that the blower is to run for five minutes prior to engine starting. (See Vapor Alarms.)

The blowers and the engines both suck air and, to some extent, are in competition. But the advantage is overwhelmingly to the engines.

Troubleshooting Fuses may blow, and brushes may wear down. In other words, the switch may be "on," but the blower may not be running. It is worthwhile each time to check for actual operation.

Lack of sufficient air at the carburetor causes the fuel mixture to the engine to become too rich, with degraded performance and economy.

NOTE: A spark-protected blower motor is far preferable, if obtainable.

VHF–FM Radios

VHF–FM (very high frequency–frequency modulation) is now the standard intercommunication method for pleasure boats. The unit has been engineered down to a size smaller than a shoebox and combines a receiver and a transmitter; in other words, it is a transceiver. Prices have moderated to a range acceptable to a boat owner.

VHF–FM RADIOS

Band	Abbreviation	Range of frequency	Range of wave length
Audio frequency	AF	20 to 20,000 cps	15,000,000 to 15,000 m
Radio frequency	RF	10 kc to 300,000 mc	30,000 m to 0.1 cm
Very low frequency	VLF	10 to 30 kc	30,000 to 10,000 m
Low frequency	LF	30 to 300 kc	10,000 to 1,000 m
Medium frequency	MF	300 to 3,000 kc	1,000 to 10 m
High frequency	HF	3 to 30 mc	100 to 10 m
Very high frequency	VHF	30 to 300 mc	10 to 1 m
Ultra high frequency	UHF	300 to 3,000 mc	100 to 10 cm
Super high frequency	SHF	3,000 to 30,000 mc	10 to 1 cm
Extremely high frequency	EHF	30,000 to 300,000 mc	1 to 0.1 cm
Heat and infrared*		10^6 to 3.9×10^6 mc	0.03 to 7.6×10^{-5} cm
Visible spectrum*		3.9×10^6 to 7.9×10^6 mc	7.6×10^{-5} to 3.8×10^{-5} cm
Ultraviolet*		7.9×10^6 to 2.3×10^{10} mc	3.8×10^{-5} to 1.3×10^{-6} cm
X-rays*		2.0×10^6 to 3.0×10^{13} mc	1.5×10^{-5} to 1.0×10^{-9} cm
Gamma rays*		2.3×10^{12} to 3.0×10^{14} mc	1.3×10^{-8} to 1.0×10^{-10} cm
Cosmic rays*		> 4.8×10^{15} mc	< 6.2×10^{-12} cm

VHF-FM RADIOS—The VHF (very high frequency) transceiver has taken over all short-range pleasure boat communication. A valuable feature of the VHF is "scanning" that automatically checks for traffic on a series of channels.

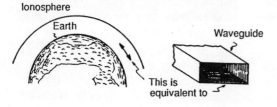

VHF-FM RADIO—The space between the Earth and the inside of the ionosphere functions like a wave guide for the passage of radio waves.

VHF-FM RADIO—High-frequency radio transmissions travel in straight lines ("line of sight").

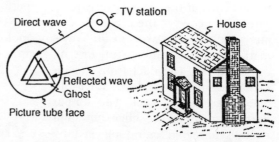

Transmitter output power is limited by law to 25 watts, providing an average communicating distance of 25 miles under good conditions.

A section of the radio spectrum, between 156 and 163 megahertz, has been set aside for exclusive VHF marine use. This has, in turn, been divided into numbered channels marked for special purposes. For example, Channel 16 is for distress and calling while general conversation is prohibited. Channels are referred to by number and not by frequency. The federal rules that govern user conduct on the channels are, in truth, technical statements of common courtesy.

A VHF transceiver is available on the market in simple, stripped-down style or more elaborate, depending on price. The lower-cost units have a limited number of channels that are accessed by a rotary switch. (Channel 16 must be included by law.) The more expensive transceivers provide all existing channels and select them digitally with telephone-type push buttons. All units must be able to switch down to 1 watt output to reduce clutter for nearby talking. All units feature a squelch control to eliminate inter-station radio noise.

A version of the VHF transceiver, scaled down in size and called a "hand-held," is much used by the dockmasters of marinas for communicating with arriving customers. The output power of a hand-held is less than 5 watts and is supplied by rechargeable internal batteries. Featured by latest model VHFs are direct dialing and scrambling for privacy.

The internal circuit of the receiver of a VHF transceiver is technically known as a "double-conversion superheterodyne." The incoming signal is heterodyned (converted) to 10.7 megahertz and then to 455 kilohertz because it is amplified more efficiently at these lower frequencies. Any one of several forms of detectors then retrieves the message for the listener. The circuit is extremely sensitive and able to process signals of even a few microvolts.

The design and construction of the antenna relieve the VHF transceiver of the need for a ground, and natural conditions provide a counterpoise. (The metal body of an automobile forms the counterpoise for the car's whip antenna.) (See Antenna.)

Modern transceivers have abandoned the quartz crystals of early models and have synthesized frequencies for both transmission and reception. This gives wider frequency range, saves space, and saves money. Fancy extras, like scanning, are now commonplace.

There are two systems by which a voice is made to "ride" a radio wave in marine service: frequency modulation (FM) and amplitude modulation (AM). With FM, the voice governs the wave frequency; with AM, the voice governs the wave amplitude.

VHF transceivers include one or more channels for weather reports.

Maintenance Maintenance of a VHF consists of wiping it clean and protecting it from spray. Checking to see whether the pilot lamp lights when the switch is on marks the limit of troubleshooting for the nontechnician. The light proves the continuity of the circuit to the battery and through the fuse. Beyond that, common sense and the law mandate licensed professional attention.

Repair Repairing the VHF requires accurate test instrumentation. Therefore, the VHF is not home-repairable.

Video Charts

Managing a paper chart while doing a trick at the wheel often seems to require a skipper endowed with three

VIDEO CHARTS

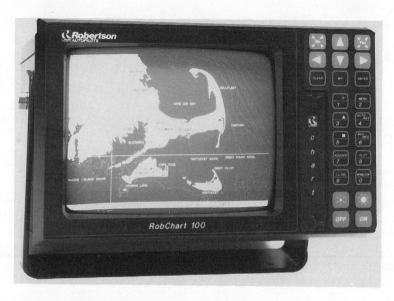

VIDEO CHARTS—The chart cartridges with which this viewer is loaded are minutely exact copies of government publications. A zoom control enlarges local details. Continuous ship's position may be shown when the needed data are fed in. *(Courtesy Robertson)*

hands. Now, along comes the video chart, which substitutes an electronic display on a console-situated screen for the paper. A zoom control allows points of interest in the picture to be enlarged. Of course, this boon requires the purchase of software cartridges, one for each area to be navigated, in place of the paper chart. The software "builds" the picture on the screen.

When navigational and speed information is added to its input, the video chart display becomes more than just a static picture; a marker maintains the boat at its true relationship with the area shown. The cartridge charts are at different scales. The viewer has the option of zooming a portion of the display in order to get better deatil, or he can call up the same area on a larger scale on another cartridge.

The video chart can lead to some effortless piloting. An example: What course to steer to reach Point A, assuming no current? Answer: Note the range and angle from the indicated position of the boat to Point A, and adapt this to the present course.

The cartridges are electronic copies of standard charts. These copies are made by the various manufacturers; there is no participation by government to assure accuracy, but quality nevertheless is high. One method of reproduction digitizes the meaningful points on the chart to supply data for the software. Another method is more like a photograph and breaks the picture into a raster like television to get software data for the cartridges. (The path the electron beam takes in composing a picture is called the "raster.")

VOLT AND AMPERE METERS

It is assumed that an official paper chart always is available for verification. One factor in the cost of cartridges and viewer is the level of detail, with the raster method at the top.

Note that the display unit of the video chart is merely a repeater that reads the software and projects the information for the convenience of the helmsman; it is not a factor in the accuracy of placement of the ship's relative position. This desirable accuracy is determined by the quality of the signals inserted by the Sat-Nav System, the Transit System, the GPS (Global Positioning System), or the Loran (see Satellite-Navigation Systems and Loran-C).

The scene on the video chart is reminiscent of radar, but in much greater detail and with a "live" rather than a shadowy appearance.

the burnout of light bulbs. This voltage regulator may be built into a metal can or it may be an internal part of some modern alternators.

The instrument voltage regulator is generally found at the back of a console meter. This regulator functions as a vibrator that selects only a portion of the line voltage, usually 5 volts. Interesting to note is that early power stations held their huge generators to correct voltage with Tyrell vibrators using the same principle.

Repair Some manufacturers recommend that voltage regulators be replaced when alternators are.

Neither regulator is repairable, though light-fingered mechanics often do some careful bending and adjusting and bring regulators back to specifications.

Voltage Regulators

The voltage in a basic alternator-to-battery connection circuit varies too widely for good battery service and far too widely if console instruments are to give meaningful readings. The difficulty arises from the nature of the alternator: Its output voltage varies with engine speed. The solution lies with a voltage regulator, one type of overall voltage control, another for the "fine tuning" needed for instruments.

The basic voltage regulator intermittently places a resistor in the alternator field circuit. This holds voltage to a safe maximum for the battery and prevents

Volt and Ampere Meters

Voltmeters and ampere meters (ammeters) are the basic tools for measuring the flow of electric current. The two are outwardly similar but internally very different. The voltmeter winding consists of many turns of fine wire, while the ammeter has very few turns of coarse wire. Also, the two meters are connected into circuits in opposite manner: Voltmeters are connected across the line, whereas ammeters are connected in series with the load. The voltmeter is a high-resistance device; the ammeter has low re-

VOLT AND AMPERE METERS

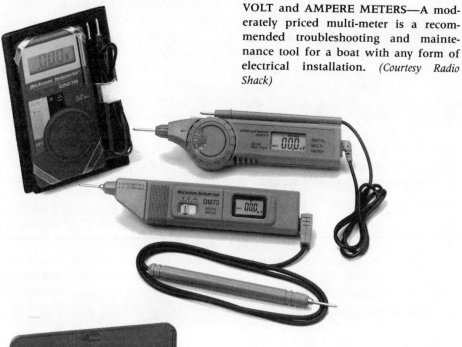

VOLT and AMPERE METERS—A moderately priced multi-meter is a recommended troubleshooting and maintenance tool for a boat with any form of electrical installation. *(Courtesy Radio Shack)*

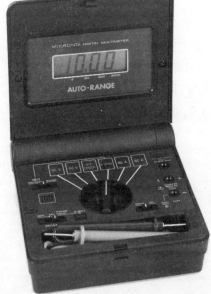

VOLT and AMPERE METERS—Three of the styles in which compact multi-meters with digital readings are available for boat use. *(Courtesy Beckman Industrial)*

sistance. Both act by responding to the magnetic field caused by the flow of the electric current to be measured.

A voltohmmeter contains a battery and switches from volts to amperes to ohms of resistance. (See Voltohmmeters.)

Less commonly in use is the watt meter (see Watt Meters). This instruments automatically combines the volts and amperes flowing in a circuit and gives the result in watts, the unit of power. (Watts over a period of time is the equivalent of work performed, and is the basis for a utility company's charges.)

Because the voltmeter contains a coil with many turns of fine copper wire, it has high resistance. This coil (actually the terminals of the meter) is *always* connected across the line. The resulting magnetism of the coil attracts an iron segment that moves the pointer over a calibrated scale to indicate the voltage of the circuit, the presence of "pressure."

The ammeter always is connected in series with the line, *never* across. This is logical, since the ammeter indicates the presence of flow. The ammeter contains the equivalent of a one-turn coil of heavy copper wire; this explains its low resistance. The reason for the low resistance is to interfere as little as possible with the flow of current. As with the voltmeter, the magnetism of the coil moves a needle across a calibrated scale. Meters are designated for direct-current and for alternating-current circuits, usually not for both, unless there is compensating circuitry.

The simple meters described above are representative of most of the instruments found on boat consoles. Laboratory meters are of a type called D'Arsonval; these are more accurate, more complex, and more expensive. Their moving-needle systems are carefully balanced and move on jeweled bearings compensated for temperature.

The most useful device for the average boat owner in dealing with his electrical system is the multimeter. Available in pocket size with a digital readout, the multimeter measures voltage in either AC or DC, resistance, diodes, and continuity—all in one compact unit.

The basic voltmeter is an all-around device widely used for measurings other than voltage. With proper calibration and in the correct circuit, the scale may read miles per hours, depth in feet, revolutions per minute, or whatever.

Troubleshooting The simplest manner in which to check the accuracy of a meter is to substitute an instrument of known fidelity and compare the readings for identical conditions. Minute bending of the spring should cause correction. Meters should not be used beyond their rating; doing so may cause error and burnout.

Voltohmmeter (VOM)

The molded case of a voltohmmeter contains a high-resistance voltmeter, a flashlight battery, a series of calibrated resistors, and a multipoint switch for connecting these items in various patterns. Two flexible leads leave the case and serve as the VOM connectors. The switch provides a number of resistance scales on the meter, from very low to very high in ohms. Several ranges are also available for pure voltage measurements of both alternating and direct currents.

By touching one meter lead to the beginning of a circuit and the other lead to the end, a reading of the circuit condition is obtained. If this reading agrees with the specifications, the circuit is in order. A very low or zero reading is the herald of a short circuit. A very high or infinity reading announces a break in the continuity—in other words, a break in the circuit.

The overriding caution with the VOM is that it must *never* be connected

WATER PURIFIERS

to any circuit containing voltage when the meter is switched to the resistance-reading mode.

The adjustment knob on the VOM is manipulated as follows: With the two leads in contact with each other and the swtich set for a resistance reading, the knob is used to set the meter needle on zero. With the leads not touching, the needle should be on infinity.

Maintenance The flashlight battery in the VOM is the only part of the instrument that requires maintenance over a period of time. The condition of this battery is judged by whether or not it is possible to achieve a zero reading, as noted above. Intervals of replacement are long because modern batteries have excellent, long shelf life and service in the VOM is only momentary. The leads should never be touched to circuits with voltages higher than the range to which the scale is set. With unknown voltages, start with the highest setting and work down to the proper range.

Water Purifiers

That old sailor's lament, "Water, water everywhere, but not a drop to drink," no longer holds true. Compact water-purifying equipment takes seawater and brings it up to a quality level sufficient for drinking. The process is automatic, removes all contaminants, and uses onboard electricity. Desalination is one of the purifier's duties. On the basis of weight, size, and power requirement, a purifying installation is well within the capability of a medium-sized yacht.

Reverse-osmosis water purification is the heart of the system in general use. (This is not a distillation process.) The osmotic cell is a spirally wound, thin film polyamide composite. It is easily cleaned without disassembling, and it is replaceable.

Seawater is rated by the number of parts per million (PPM) of dissolved solids it contains and by its acidity (pH). The solids are removed by several stages of filtration that stop particles as small as approximately 10 microns. Separators prevent oil contamination of the osmotic membrane. The entire system may be cleaned by simple reverse flushing between duty cycles. Some units automatically reject output water that is below drinking quality. This requires a salt residue less than approximately 1 percent, when seawater is the input.

"Osmosis" is the natural tendency toward equalization that occurs when two liquids of unequal concentration are separated by a partially permeable diaphragm. The membrane itself, acting as a filter, removes more than 98 percent of the minerals dissolved in the water to be purified.

Maintenance Flow meters and pressure gauges in the installation keep track of the need for cleanout by reverse flushing, and supply information on which to judge the need for osmosis cartridge replacement.

Troubleshooting Troubleshooting is a step-by-step analysis from input to output and a check on the operation of the pumps.

Repair None of the components is repairable, only replaceable.

Water Tanks

Water in the storage tank(s) aboard a boat is heavy and takes its toll in fuel and speed. Hence, it is generally bad economy to fill the water tank(s) for a one-day cruise; take only an appropriate amount for the day. (There is a caution here, however: Some boats require the ballasting effect of a full water tank or tanks to trim and ride best.)

Installation A popular location for a water tank is under a berth. When this berth is far off longitudinal center, it may be necessary to pair it with a duplicate tank an equal distance on the other side of center in order to avert a list. The two are connected by a pipe or hose (see Hose Safety) for equalization. (In choosing tank capacity, remember that weight is the enemy of the boat's performance.) A flange-type fill plate on the outer deck is a necessary convenience. The tanks should contain baffles to prevent noisy sloshing. More or less complex tank gauges are available.

A breather vent is important; without it, the vacuum caused by water being drawn off will collapse the tank.

Maintenance The water tank on a boat run only on weekends is subject to a very low frequency of use, and it becomes a likely candidate for bacterial infection. The antidote is the chlorine in household bleach. The procedure is to superchlorinate and then to dechlorinate the water that is to be used. This applies to all boat water tanks, be they of lined wood, plastic, or metal.

The household bleach is added at the rate of approximately one teaspoon to one tablespoon per gallon, depending on local condition and the source of the water. (A high degree of chlorination is safer and not objectionable because of subsequent dechlorination.) Chlorination is a recommended procedure regardless of the water source because it also keeps protecting the tank.

The recommended routine for dechlorination is to boil enough water to fill a large bottle and then to keep this in the refrigerator for drinking. (The boiling is only momentary, to dispel the chlorine.) Water for cooking is placed on the stove and allowed to boil before food ingredients are added.

The foregoing steps not only protect against dangerous drinking water—they sanitize the tank as well. Many mates add a few drops of lemon or lime juice per glass of water to improve flavor.

Watt Meters

A radio-frequency watt meter indicates the actual power being generated by a VHF transceiver without regard to the percentage of it that is usefully being radiated by the antenna. This is in contrast to the SWR meter that indicates antenna circuit efficiency without regard to the amount of power flowing (see Standing Wave Ratio).

The watt meter is connected in series with the lead from the transceiver to the antenna by means of standard coax connectors. ("Series" means that the meter is "cut" into the line between transmitter and antenna, and the power runs through it.) The meter will

WEATHER

give a reading whenever, and as long as, the push-to-talk button is pressed. The correct watt meter is selected on the basis of transceiver output, for instance, 25-watt range (or slightly above) for a VHF.

The watt meter needle soon becomes a subconsciously watched telltale of radio condition. A steep drop is the red flag of trouble. The quiver of the needle in relation to talk into the microphone is an indication of the modulation.

With cost in mind, very few transceiver installations incorporate an output power meter. A substitute for the meter is a small red bulb that glows during transmissions. The intensity of the glow is a rough indication of the power.

(NOTE: One watt is equal to one ampere times one volt; see Electricity, Volt and Ampere Meters.)

Weather

The wind brings the weather. An observant skipper unconsciously totals and catalogs his experiences and soon becomes his own local weather forecaster. As an all-around backup and final word, there are the official government stations continuously broadcasting weather information on VHF radio.

Weather forecasting is under the auspices of the National Oceanic and Atmospheric Administration (NOAA). A chain of broadcasting stations makes radio reception available in almost all boating areas. The various transmitting frequencies are grouped just above 162 megahertz, and the installations are known as WX-1, WX-2, WX-3, etc. All VHF transceivers make provision for receiving weather.

Weather is a huge heat engine that never stops running. Air is warmed and rises. Cooler air enters the consequently lower-pressure areas. Air motions (winds) are formed that often bring moisture and may be deviated by the rotation of the Earth. Cooling condenses the moisture into rain. Air arriving from a cold region (cold front) often mingles with air from a warm region (warm front) to cause local bad weather. All these local happenings are the reason why local observations must "shade" the information from the NOAA stations, in order to be most helpful.

Clouds also form and speak a "language" of their own in passing on weather information to the initiated skipper who can decipher them. The most infamous cloud, from the pleasure boater's point of view, is the forbidding cumulonimbus with its giant, dark anvil that portends a lightning storm, usually with little advance warning (see Lightning).

Fog, most feared of obstructions to marine sight, is a cloud low enough to touch the earth. A mass of air containing moisture has been cooled enough to cause partial condensation into tiny droplets that block sight. Usually, the sun disperses fog by revaporizing the droplets; in boat talk, the fog "burns off." (See Cruising Hazards.)

The amount of moisture air can hold is proportional to its temperature; the cooler the air, the less moisture. When

WEATHER

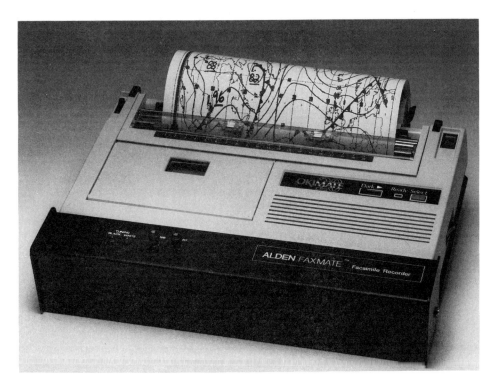

WEATHER—The wonders of radio facsimile (fax) transmission can place an up-to-the-minute weather map in the hands of the cruising skipper regardless of where his course takes him. Fifty stations around the world broadcast this information. In addition, he receives printed messages on safety and other subjects.

Facsimile, weather, safety, and teletype broadcasts take place on frequencies between 100 kilohertz and 30 megahertz. Weather chart recorders are available that self-tune to these radio bands or else hook onto equivalent radio receivers already aboard.

Shown is a popular weather chart recorder. Operation is automatic once the correct signal is fed in. Start and stop commands are contained in the weather transmission.

A bonus with this instrument is that it may be used as the printer for a computer. *(Courtesy Alden Electronics)*

the moisture content for a given temperature is at its maximum, the air is said to be "saturated," and its relative humidity is 100 percent. Supersaturation is possible under certain conditions.

The various boating areas of the country have their own unique weather problems and breed cautions that soon impress themselves upon local skippers. Thus, Florida has the possibility of hurricanes from June through November, and effective alert systems keep boaters from forgetting. Unusual bad weather in the form of wind and fog is related to the calendar in other places, and the warning is subconsciously ever present.

An AM radio emits crackles and bangs well in advance of the arrival of a lightning storm. (A correctly adjusted FM radio does not respond to this electrical noise and is of no use as a warning.)

The information available from NOAA radio broadcasts is greatly amplified by weather maps. These maps are printed in newspapers, are shown on TV, and—latest wonder of wonders—they may be produced right on the boat with radio facsimile equipment. Standardized symbols and abbreviations on the maps convey inordinate amounts of data relative to wind, barometric pressure, precipitation, humidity, temperature, fronts, etc., at a given station.

Sound takes approximately 5 seconds to travel 1 mile, and this provides a rule-of-thumb distance calculator for lightning. The one-and, two-and, three-and style of counting one second per digit is begun at the instant of the lightning flash, and ended with the sound of thunder. The total count, divided by 5, is the distance in miles to the site of the lightning. A series of declining counts means that the lightning is getting closer.

Wind is named for the direction *from* which it blows. Wind speed may be expressed in simple miles per hour, in knots, in kilometers per hour, or by a number of the Beaufort Scale. (Beaufort 0 designates calm; Beaufort 12 is the equivalent of 64 knots.) A wind changing direction in a clockwise direction is "veering"; if in a counterclockwise direction, it is "backing."

Instruments for measuring wind velocity range from primitive to complex. Simplest is a calibrated transparent tube containing a pith ball. The tube is held in the wind so that the air passing over the open end creates a suction that raises the ball to a reading. The more serious devices contain wind-actuated propellers or paddles whose revolutions per minute are read on a scale as wind speed. Another measuring type makes use of a Pitot tube and meter, much as is done on airplanes.

The boatman underway deals with two kinds of wind: the true wind and the apparent wind. The telltale on the mast, or a burgee, shows the apparent wind, a vectored combination of Nature's wind and the wind caused by the forward motion of the boat. (See Vectors.)

Winches

A winch is a mechanism that applies mechanical advantages to multiply the force a person can exert to reel in a line. The terms "windlass," "capstan," and "winch" are often used interchangeably, although this is not strictly "according to the book." Some claim that a winch with a vertical drum is a capstan, although most modern halyard and sheet winches have vertical drums. Some winches have handles that turn or ratchet through only a part of a turn, while other handles turn full circle like the "coffee grinders" so often mentioned during *America*'s Cup races. The foregoing winches are all

WINCHES

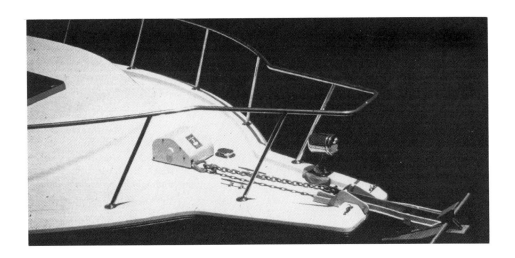

WINCHES—Shown is a complete bow installation for efficient anchoring. In addition to the winch, there is the pulpit and the bow roller. *(Courtesy Powerwinch)*

manually operated and are found only on sailboats for handling the running rigging.

Powerboats also make use of winches but carry only one that is power-operated and devoted exclusively to anchor handling. A sailboat may also carry such a power winch for anchoring. A similar winch may also be found on trailers to help in launching and retrieving boats. The power to operate these winches is drawn from the 12-volt storage battery.

A word on terminology: A winch drum with a smooth surface for handling line is a "gypsy." A drum with a machined surface designed to accommodate chain is a "wildcat." Maintaining tension on the line coming off the drum, to avoid slippage, is "tailing."

The manual winches multiply the human force expended upon them by a ratio determined by the winch gearing. For instance, 50 pounds on the winch handle results in a 1,000-pound pull on the halyard or sheet when the ratio is 20 to 1 and friction is assumed to be the impossible zero. This does not signify a free bonus from Nature; Nature gives nothing for nothing. What has happened is that the input has traveled 20 times as far as the output in order to balance the equation. (Had that been a two-stage 20-to-1 winch, the mechanical advantage would have been at least double.)

The electrically operated anchor and trailer winches turn battery power into pulling power. They can achieve great pulling power without ruinous battery drains by running the small motor very fast and the hauling drum very slow. (Again, nothing for nothing.) This relationship of small, high-speed, low-current motor and slow-speed hauling drum has enabled one manufacturer to introduce a cordless trailer winch that contains a rechargeable battery.

A good sailboat winch is a precision-made mechanism and a thing of beauty, but its handle may become a lethal object if a "dog" (or brake) gives way under load and the handle flies off. (The handle should never be left in the winch.)

Winches intended for installation on deck to help with the anchor feed the incoming rode directly into the rope locker. They are controlled by a remote switch. The smaller units are battery-powered, while the larger models are wired into the high-voltage system on boats with generators. An improvement in anchor winches is the "free fall" feature of the winch that allows the anchor to drop without hindrance to assure a better grip on the bottom.

Self-tailing winches eliminate the need for manually keeping the line tight around the drum. Many winches are now designed as the main components within automatic anchoring units. These units handle the anchor rode, both up and down, in response to electric push buttons at the console, without manual aid; some also indicate rode length in feet as a help in safe anchoring.

Maintenance The maintenance of winches for the running rigging concerns itself with appearance, lubrication, and wear. It is a natural impulse for a sailor proud of his boat to polish and shine a beautiful object of aluminum or bronze on his deck. More practically, winch manufacturers recommend frequent lubrication and periodic inspection. It is questionable whether unskilled hands should dismantle gearing originally installed to an accuracy of one-thousandth of an inch. Lubrication should be with a grease approved by the winch maker and usually supplied in handy squeeze tubes.

The internal parts to inspect closely for wear are the ratchet and its dog. The strain on the dog is great, and its tip may be developing a roundness that can lead to failure. As mentioned earlier, a dog suddenly giving up its ghost may lead to serious trouble.

Maintenance kits of spare parts are available to aid in performing the recommended inspection and necessary replacement. These kits contain pawls, retaining rings, cotter pins, washers, and cap screws. It is assumed that the simple tools found aboard will do the job.

Repair A well-made and well-designed winch from a good manufacturer should go into ripe old age without needing more than the maintenance kit supplies. When trouble goes deeper than that, it is time for the professionals. Installing gears so that the teeth mesh exactly according to the book takes know-how and experience. Inaccuracy grinds gear teeth down quickly in use.

Wind/Current vs. Course

The direction in which wind and current tend to push the boat may be at variance with the skipper's chosen course. Consequently, he must be able to judge the amount and direction of the forces he must apply to counteract Nature.

Hulls and superstructures of powerboats and sailboats differ, and it is logical to expect their reactions to wind

WIRE ROPE

WIRE ROPE—Wire rope is preferred by racing skippers for the standing rigging of their sailboats. The 6 x 19, in various diameters, is widely used.

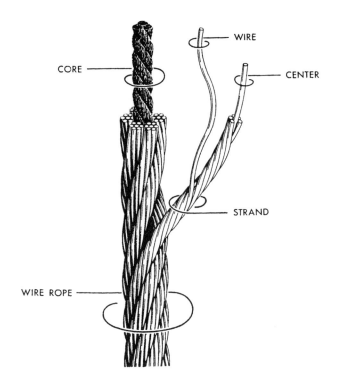

and current to differ. Powerboats have large exposure to wind and relatively small immersed surface available to the current; furthermore, their bow-on, stern-on, and broad-on exposures differ in the amount of Nature's energy these surfaces will absorb. Sailboats also present such variations, but a greater portion of hull is immersed, making sailboarts more sensitive to current.

These offsetting forces are taken into account when plotting a course; they are "vectored" in (see Plotting, Vectors). Much similar vectoring may be done mentally when piloting. The wind and current are imagined as arrows whose length coincides with the opposing tide or current and whose angles relative to the boat are actual. The mental picture now becomes a connected series of arrows whose resultant vector (the third side of the "triangle") is readily approximated to find the necessary action.

Wire Rope

Wire rope is preferred for the standing rigging of sailboats, especially if they are racing craft. The advantages of wire rope over synthetic fiber are greater strength, less stretch, and, with modern alloy wire, longer life span. (The alloys have supplanted the more common zinc-coated galvanized-base wire for critical installations.)

WIRE SPLICES

The wire for rope is drawn from heat-treated rod. The wire is preformed and then shaped into strands. The strands are wound about a cored or coreless center to form the rope, and the direction of winding becomes a "left lay" or a "right lay." The direction of lay is a critical factor in the use of the rope.

Wire rope is specified by two numbers in addition to its diameter, as, for instance, 6 × 19. The first digit is the number of strands—in this case, six. A bit of confusion enters with the second digits, because the number of wires per strand may be as many as 25. The core may be a wire, a plastic rod, natural fiber, or the rope may be coreless, as noted above.

Maintenance Wire rope needs lubrication with a lube oil that is not too thin and has sticking and penetrating power.

Troubleshooting Wire rope is sensitive to the equipment with which it is used. Sheave jaws should fit the wire. Too large an opening robs the wire of support; too small subjects the wire to undesirable crushing.

A frequent cause of wear in wire rope is a lack of alignment of sheaves, causing rubbing within the blocks. Another is blocks too small with undersize sheaves that cause sharp reverse bends.

Wire Splices

One of the most effective methods of joining two current-carrying electric wires has been around since the early days of the telegraph and is appropriately named the "Western Union splice." This splice has great tensile strength and low resistance, even without soldering.

The insulation of both wires is stripped off for about 1 inch. The two bare wires then are crossed at midpoint and given two twists about each other. The two remaining bare sections are then coiled tightly about the adjacent bare wire in the space left before the insulation.

The central twist provides tensile strength. The tight coiling reduces electrical resistance. Shining copper is mandatory if soldering follows (see Soldering).

Total insulation is restored with electrical tape in the usual manner.

Wiring Code

The American Boat & Yacht Council has developed an identifying color code for the electric wiring aboard a pleasure boat. This makes it easy to pick a desired circuit from a bundle of wires when repair or replacement makes it necessary. The coding is achieved by using wires with insula-

WIRING CODE—This table of electrical copper wire weights and resistances should enable more accurate purchase and use when installations or alterations are proposed. These specifications are an aid in selecting the proper wire carrying capacity for a given load. *(Courtesy ABYC)*

WIRING CODE

Gage No.	Diameter in mils at 20 deg. cent.	Pounds per 1,000 ft.	Feet per pound	Feet per Ohm* 20 deg. cent. (= 68 deg. fahr.)	Feet per Ohm* 50 deg. cent. (= 122 deg. fahr.)
0000	460.0	640.5	1.561	20,400.0	18,250.0
000	409.6	507.9	1.968	16,180.0	14,470.0
00	364.8	402.8	2.482	12,830.0	11,480.0
0	324.9	319.5	3.130	10,180.0	9,103.0
1	289.3	253.3	3.947	8,070.0	7,219.0
2	257.6	200.9	4.977	6,400.0	5,725.0
3	229.4	159.3	6.276	5,075.0	4,540.0
4	204.3	126.4	7.914	4,025.0	3,600.0
5	181.9	100.2	9.980	3,192.0	2,855.0
6	162.0	79.46	12.58	2,531.0	2,264.0
7	144.3	63.02	15.87	2,007.0	1,796.0
8	128.5	49.98	20.01	1,592.0	1,424.0
9	114.4	39.63	25.23	1,262.0	1,129.0
10	101.9	31.43	31.82	1,001.0	895.6
11	90.74	24.92	40.12	794.0	710.2
12	80.81	19.77	50.59	629.6	563.2
13	71.96	15.68	63.80	499.3	446.7
14	64.08	12.43	80.44	396.0	354.2
15	57.07	9.858	101.4	314.0	280.9
16	50.82	7.818	127.9	249.0	222.8
17	45.26	6.200	161.3	197.5	176.7
18	40.30	4.917	203.4	156.6	140.1
19	35.89	3.899	256.5	124.2	111.1
20	31.96	3.092	323.4	98.50	88.11
21	28.46	2.452	407.8	78.11	69.87
22	25.35	1.945	514.2	61.95	55.41
23	22.57	1.542	648.4	49.13	43.94
24	20.10	1.223	817.7	38.96	34.85
25	17.90	0.9699	1,031.0	30.90	27.64
26	15.94	0.7692	1,300.0	24.50	21.92
27	14.20	0.6100	1,639.0	19.43	17.38
28	12.64	0.4837	2,067.0	15.41	13.78
29	11.26	0.3836	2,607.0	12.22	10.93
30	10.03	0.3042	3,287.0	9.691	8.669
31	8.928	0.2413	4,145.0	7.685	6.875
32	7.950	0.1913	5,227.0	6.095	5.452
33	7.080	0.1517	6,591.0	4.833	4.323
34	6.305	0.1203	8,310.0	3.833	3.429
35	5.615	0.09542	10,480.0	3.040	2.719
36	5.000	0.07568	13,210.0	2.411	2.156
37	4.453	0.06001	16,660.0	1.912	1.710
38	3.965	0.04759	21,010.0	1.516	1.356
39	3.531	0.03774	26,500.0	1.202	1.075
40	3.145	0.02993	33,410.0	0.9534	0.8529

*Length at 20 deg. cent. of a wire whose resistance is 1 ohm at the stated temperatures.

WIRING CODE

RECOMMENDED MARINE WIRING COLOR CODE
DIRECT CURRENT SYSTEMS — UNDER 50 VOLTS

COLOR	ITEM	USE
Yellow w/Red Stripe (YR)	Starting Circuit	Starting Switch to Solenoid
Yellow (Y)	Generator or Alternator Field	Generator or Alternator Field to Regulator Field Terminal
	Bilge Blowers	Fuse or Switch to Blowers
Dark Gray (Gy)	Navigation Lights	Fuse or Switch to Lights
	Tachometer	Tachometer Sender to Gauge
Brown (Br)	Generator Armature	Generator Armature to Regulator
	Alternator Charge Light	Generator Terminal/Alternator Auxiliary Terminal to Light to Regulator
	Pumps	Fuse or Switch to Pumps
Orange (O)	Accessory Feed	Ammeter to Alternator or Generator Output and Accessory Fuses or Switches
	Accessory Common Feed	Distribution Panel to Accesory Switch
Purple (Pu)	Ignition	Ignition Switch to Coil and Electrical Instruments
	Instrument Feed	Distribution Panel to Electric Instruments
Dark Blue	Cabin and Instrument Lights	Fuse or Switch to Lights
Light Blue (Lt Bl)	Oil Pressure	Oil Pressure Sender to Gauge
Tan	Water Temperature	Water Temperature Sender to Gauge
Pink (Pk)	Fuel Gauge	Fuel Gauge Sender to Gauge

WIRING CODE—Holding all boat wiring to this standardized color code makes subsequent troubleshooting easier.

INSTALLATION CAUTIONS:
- When AC and DC conductors are run together in a common trough, tube, or raceway, the AC conductors shall be loomed or jacketed separately from the DC conductors.
- Color coding may be used on systems wired with one-color insulation by utilizing appropriately colored sleeving or by other permanent means of applying color to all wiring termination points.

Where numerals, letters, color coding, or other identification is applied by any form of tape wrapped around the conductor, the tape shall have a minimum width of 3/16 inch, shall have sufficient length to make at least two complete turns around the conductor, and shall be visible near each terminal. *(Courtesy American Boat & Yacht Council)*

tion of assorted colors. Coding may also be done with colored plastic tape encircling the wire near its end. (Any of these coding systems is less bother than actual labeling.)

The ABYC rules cover the wiring for direct current of 50 volts or less, such as usually supplied by batteries. Contrary to shoreside electrical codes, low-voltage DC and high-voltage AC wirings may be run in the same trough if they are not bundled together.

The ABYC classifies conductors (wires) as follows: A "bonding conductor" carries no current and bonds all metal housings, etc. to the boat's safety bonding system. A "grounded conductor" carries current and is usually negative. A "grounding conductor" carries no current and prevents shocks by connecting equipment enclosures to ground. An "ungrounded conductor" is the "hot" wire from the source of power, usually the positive pole of the battery.

All insulated grounding conductors shall be green. (If these wires are uninsulated, they need no identification.) The colors green and white are *not* to be used for ungrounded, current-carrying conductors. Three-wire alternating-current cables are to use black, white, and red; four-wire systems are restricted to black, white, red, and blue.

There is an overall release in the ABYC code: A system of individual choice may be substituted for the color code if a complete wiring diagram is provided.

Routine inspection of wiring is recommended, because the marine environment is the number-one enemy of low-resistance electrical connections. Beware of the green encrustation of corrosion!

Zincs

Every skipper who has metal attached to the bottom of his hull knows zinc, both from his pocketbook and from the trouble of maintaining zincs in active condition. But, in truth, zinc is not a one-way expense, although it may appear to be so. The money necessarily spent on zinc is returned as a saving on props, skegs, shafts, and whatever other metal components must be down there.

Zinc is number two in the electrolytic activity of metals, and far more active than the bronzes, etc., normally found in marine usage. Thus, zinc sacrifices itself to protect the other metals to which it is connected and with which it is submerged. Zinc is the "sacrificial anode." (See Electrolysis.)

Zincs are available in many shapes and sizes, and suppliers maintain large sheets from which to cut larger-than-standard surfaces. Collars are sold for many diameters of shafts. Most marine engines have provision for a zinc rod in the cooling system.

Installation The anode must retain full contact with the water acting as electrolyte, and therefore may not be painted, because that would provide insulation. The anode must have good electrical connection with each of the metal units it is to protect. The dissipation of the anode in a properly bal-

ZINCS

anced circuit is gradual. Unfortunately, choosing the optimum amount of zinc for a given boat is a guessing game.

Maintenance Maintenance of a zinc anode consists of keeping the zinc clean, even wirebrushing it when needed, and checking for good electrical contacts. Zinc wearing is a sign that it is doing its job. Impure zinc will remain. (The zinc for anodes is of high purity; junkyard pickups will not do.) Zincs that are badly eroded should be discarded.

Troubleshooting The familiar boast "My zincs last forever" is an admission that the zinc is not electrically connected to the circuit, and is not protecting. The weak links in the protective system are the bonding connections. These should be inspected for corrosion at every opportunity. (Screws needed for attaching zincs should be bronze.)